Manual for Effective Community Health Nursing Practice

ABOUT THE AUTHOR

Marie-Luise Friedemann (RN, BSN, MSN, Wayne State University and University of Michigan, School of Nursing) is an instructor in Psychiatric Nursing and Community Health Nursing at Eastern Michigan University. She is a doctoral candidate at the School of Education, University of Michigan.

OTHER IMPORTANT TITLES

Community Health Nursing, Second Edition by Archer & Fleshman

Understanding and Responding: A Communications Manual for Nurses by Long & Prophit

Basic Steps in Planning Nursing Research, Second Edition by Brink & Wood

Working with the Elderly: Group Process and Techniques by Irene Mortenson Burnside

Life-Cycle Group Work in Nursing by Janosik & Phipps

Ethics and Law in Nursing by Fenner

Primary Care Nursing: Crisis Model in Client Management by Thibodeau & Hawkins

MANUAL FOR EFFECTIVE COMMUNITY HEALTH NURSING PRACTICE

MARIE-LUISE FRIEDEMANN, RN, BSN, MSN
Eastern Michigan University, Ypsilanti

 WADSWORTH HEALTH SCIENCES DIVISION • Monterey, California

Subject Editor: *Adrian Perenon*
Production: *Brian Williams/San Francisco*
Manuscript Editor: *Brian Williams*
Interior Design and Photo Research: *Wendy Calmenson*
Cover Design: *Albert Burkhardt*
Illustrations: *Carl Brown*
Typesetting: *Graphic Typesetting Service, Los Angeles*
Production Services Manager: *Stacey C. Sawyer*

Wadsworth Health Sciences Division
A Division of Wadsworth, Inc.

Printed in the United States of America

10 9 8 7 6 5 4 3 2 1

ISBN 0-534-01240-X

Library of Congress Cataloging in Publication data:
Friedemann, Marie-Luise
  Manual for effective community health nursing practice

  Bibliography: p.
  Includes index.
  1. Community health nursing.   I. Title.
[DNLM: 1. Community health nursing. 2. Nursing process.
WY 106 F899m]
RT98.F74 1983   610.73′43   82-20188
ISBN 0-534-01240-X

Preface

PURPOSE

This book for nursing students has four purposes. The first is to answer questions students have about the usefulness of community health nursing in home visits and other settings. Many students come to the subject of community health nursing with the belief that it is less important and less exciting than "real" nursing—the kind that takes place in emergency rooms and intensive care units, where nursing the acutely ill patient is often a matter of life or death. In addition, students often find that the idea of home visits, which are so much a part of community health nursing, produces much anxiety: Why should they be forced to intrude into strangers' homes? I hope this book will enable students to recognize the value of home visits and help them to overcome anxiety by teaching them to look at each situation realistically and instilling confidence in their abilities.

The second purpose of the book is to introduce a simple approach to community nursing, a way to proceed with assessment and planning, and the implementation and evaluation of care. This purpose buttresses the first one, for a student who understands the procedure to follow during community nursing situations will feel confident.

The third purpose is to show the excitement of community health nursing. Not all community nursing is home visits, and not all home visits are just checking clients recently discharged from the hospital. In acute care nursing, the nurse acts largely as the executor of a medical regimen, but the community health nurse has a more independent and challenging role, acting as a part of the health promotion and maintenance systems of the community in which the client lives. Community health nurses are not only direct-care providers but also planners, organizers, and coordinators. Their role is exciting because it asks for creativity and resourcefulness. Because nurses often act without the assistance of other members of a health team, knowledge of theory—often perceived as uninteresting and impractical by students—becomes vital to them. In this book I have attempted to help students by selecting only theory that is useful and translating it into theory-based nursing actions.

The fourth purpose is to give the student practical, step-by-step guidelines for the nursing process. It suggests areas to cover and questions to ask when assessing and teaching in primary, secondary, and tertiary prevention, thus clarifying the community health nursing role to the student and thereby, I hope, increasing the student's confidence.

ORGANIZATION

The book has been organized into four parts. Part I, "Background for Community-Focused Care," takes the reader through the nursing process. Chapter 1, on assessment, describes different areas affecting the client's health and stresses the importance of promoting good health and preventing disease rather than simply concentrating on illness. The example of Robert Fox shows how different aspects in the client's life and his surroundings influence his health. The details are intended to convey a thorough understanding of the client's situation, lifestyle, support system, and so on, thereby yielding insight into the network of factors shaping his personality, interaction patterns, and physical and emotional strengths and problems.

Chapter 2 concerns the planning of care. It gives an example of how to categorize and organize problems and strengths and plan effective care. I have deliberately made the approach more detailed than community nurses are apt to have time for in reality in order to give students a feel for the complexity of holistic nursing care. With experience, nurses learn to assess and analyze many aspects in a client's situation without writing them down in the detail shown here.

Chapter 3 explains the importance of implementing and evaluating nursing care for individual clients as well as for the nursing agency as a whole. The use of records for evaluation purposes is also discussed.

Part II, "Patient Teaching for Self-Care," outlines health teaching needs in primary, secondary, and tertiary prevention. Chapters 4 through 6 offer a guide to areas affecting a client's lifestyle and health that should be covered when a nurse is giving care in the community setting. Teaching areas are listed in tables together with sample questions in order to help the nurse assess a client's knowledge and present health practices.

Part III, "Communication and Behavioral Dimensions of Community Nursing," consists of three chapters. Chapter 7 discusses the initial contact—the psycho-social and emotional aspects and problems often encountered in the beginning by nurses doing home visits. The chapter describes ways to deal with anxiety and insecurity and establish an effective nurse/client relationship.

Chapter 8, which deals with crisis intervention, gives examples of types of crisis and nursing action in order to help the student be mentally prepared for dealing with intense situations.

Chapter 9 introduces the student to practical aspects of communication techniques, the helping relationship, and teaching/learning techniques, showing how to teach the material discussed in Part II. The importance of maintaining an effective nurse/client relationship and of using empathy and communication to change a client's health behavior are stressed.

Part IV, "The Family," helps the student address clients' problems by encouraging them to think about the systems within which clients function, the influences inside and outside the family that shape their health behavior, and the behaviors and values within the family. Chapter 10 describes the individual within family and community systems. Chapter 11 discusses family interaction patterns. Chapter 12 covers aspects of the family life span and types of family encountered today. The aim of these chapters is to promote understanding of the dynamics of families and to build a foundation for comprehensive family nursing care.

USE

This book may be used in a variety of ways: (1) as a complementary text in basic, undergraduate nursing-fundamentals courses to help students prepare for clinical experiences focused on home visits; (2) for the community health nursing course, which comprises home visits as clinical training; (3) for the beginning practitioner in community health nursing or for the experienced nurse practitioner shifting to community-based service.

In closing, I would like to thank my husband, Heinrich, and my children, Karin, Stefan, and Christina, for their support and understanding during the time I was working on this *Manual for Effective Community Health Nursing Practice.*

Marie-Luise Friedemann

Contents

Introduction

Community health nursing used to be understood as the nursing care provided by public health agencies. Today, however, health professionals see it as community-focused nursing care, practiced in different types of settings. Such settings—hospitals, clinics, doctors' offices, private nursing practices, industrial clinics, schools, or the clients' homes—are integrated parts of a community. Some agencies are health resources of small communities. Others, such as large medical centers, represent a catchment area of several cities or even states.

Nurses practicing community health nursing in any of these settings need to be committed to a special cause: the promotion of health and happiness in life. With their education, nurses are in a position to help people whose circumstances may be less conducive than their own to learning about this health and happiness. The community health nurse must perceive that the client is an individual or family struggling to achieve a life that leads to the greatest emotional fulfillment and physical health possible under the circumstances.

All people have personal resources to achieve health. At times, however, these resources are paralyzed by multiple stress factors, resulting in illness or hopelessness. The community nurse attempts to recover these resources and to mobilize the client to strive toward health. Knowing that every life is a struggle toward the better, the nurse may be able to look on the client as an equal and appreciate the client's basic longing for, and moral right to, health and happiness. The only differences consist of personal factors—family and community influences that have shaped and modified the course of life from birth on.

Currents of life, however, are rather complicated, and most professionals have difficulty understanding causal relationships between variables that influence who a person is and the behavior he or she exhibits. Thus, community nurses need to examine theories, concepts, and paradigms and decide how they are useful in complementing basic understanding of life and the client's problems. For example, systems theory may give us a way of looking at clients as an integral part of the universe, a system within systems, and as individuals exchanging energy and information with the environment. "OLOF" (Optimum Level Of Functioning) or "holistic health" are two other useful concepts that can be incorporated in community nursing care. Over time, new theories emerge that enable one to view problems from different angles.

For community nursing students, then, theory is not simply a necessary evil, to be dealt with in order to pass exams. Instead, they should pick out the parts of theory which make sense to them, internalize them in their way of thinking about clients, and actually apply them. At the same time, students should keep their eyes open to the fact that life is a unique teacher that enables us to conduct our own experiments in mastering tasks, coping with difficulties, experiencing health and illness, forming friendships, or overcoming sadness. Bringing theory together with true living and experiencing creates the exciting challenge of community nursing.

The following chapters lean heavily on life experiences, yet they also use theory to explain human phenomena. However, the explanations presented in this book do not, of course, claim to be the only true way of looking at health or illness. They merely suggest to the beginner ways of incorporating theory and using it creatively.

Manual for Effective Community Health Nursing Practice

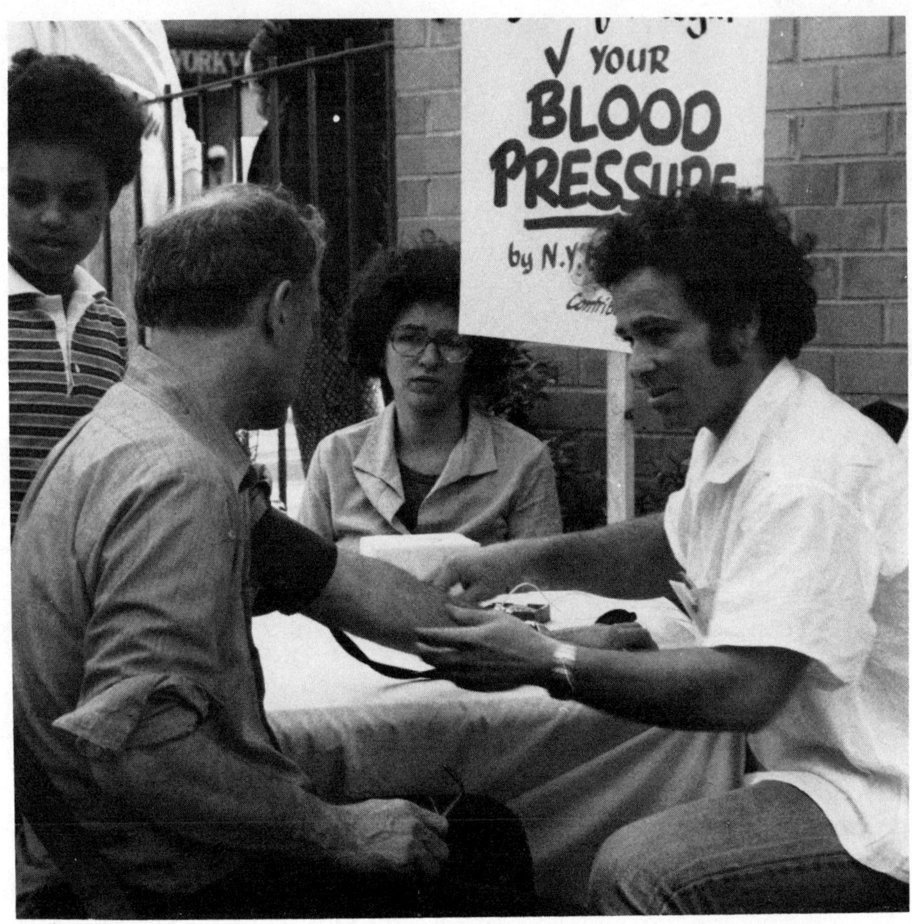

ERIKA STONE. © PETER ARNOLD, INC.

I

Background for Community-Focused Care

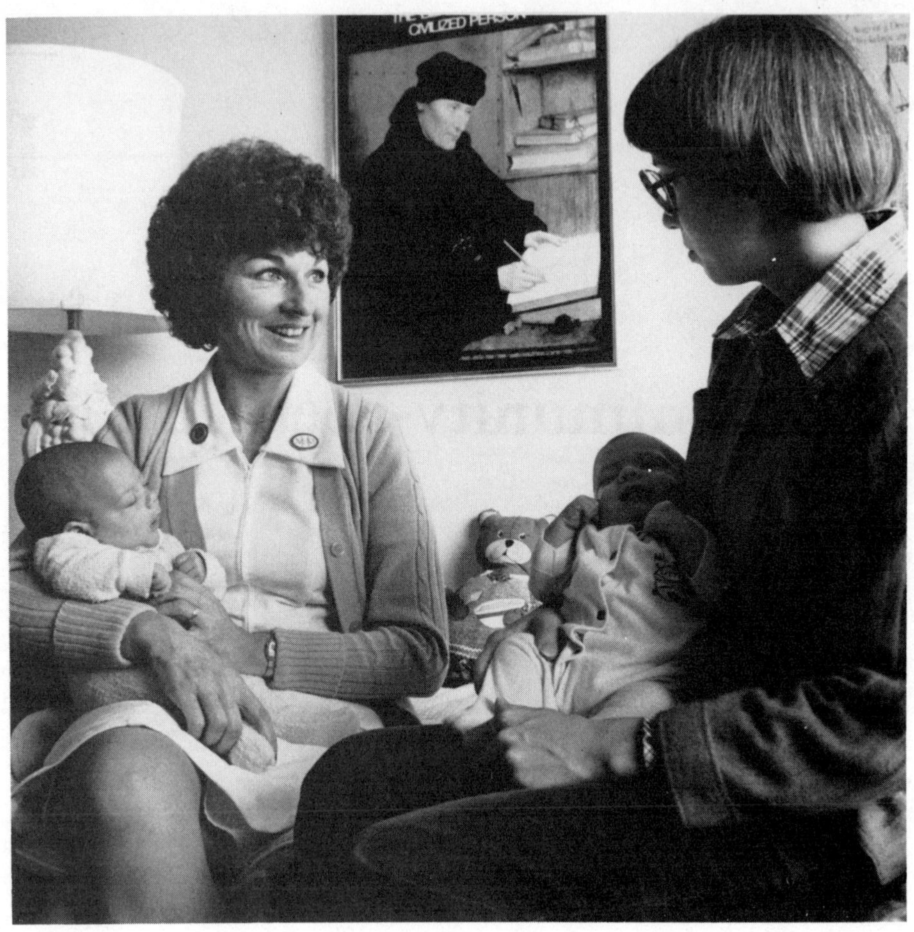

SUZANNE ARMS, © 1979

1

Assessment

Assessment is the first step in all nursing care. However, the assessment in community nursing differs from that done in hospitals, for it is concerned not only with problems of disease and comfort of the client but also with the client's individual needs as a family member and as part of the community. Moreover, assessment must also take into account all family members and others who significantly influence and are influenced by the client's life. Consequently, in community nursing we must look at a total system—the network of individuals within the family and the family within the community.

The difference in assessment, then, is the difference in looking at clients in the context of their environment. In a hospital, the client environment is rather stable and the routine of daily living is structured. Breakfast, lunch, and dinner are served at regular times, visiting hours are set, clean linen is brought to the unit at regular hours, and so on. Hospital clients have minimal influence on their environment. They need to surrender to its forces and put up with 5 AM temperature taking and flashlights in their eyes at midnight. They have to acquire a new identity in order to adapt to the hospital environment. As a result, the environment is not given the attention it deserves in planning comprehensive care.

In community health nursing, by contrast, the client environment is usually not previously known to the nurse. That environment includes social systems such as family, school, and work relationships; physical factors such as the neighborhood, work setting, home, garden, and transportation; and factors that may significantly influence a client's life from outside community limits, such as the economic situation of the state, energy shortage and cost of heating oil, industrial waste disposal, and government decisions regarding social programs. The social sciences are in agreement about the importance of the environment in determining to a large extent who people are and why they behave as they do. Thus, in order to answer the questions, Who is the client? How does he or she function and why?, the community health nurse needs to put much emphasis on the environment.

In short, the community nurse must perceive the client as an *individual*—a system with different organ parts that can be evaluated with a physical assessment, and mental-emotional subsystem that is interdependent with the organ systems which can be evaluated with a mental health assessment. In addition, because the client does not operate independently but is part of the family unit, there must be a second assessment—the *family assessment* of the client's and other family members' roles, interpersonal relationships, and communication patterns. The aim of this assessment is to pinpoint positive and negative factors that may influence the client's and other family members' well-being and self-perception. Finally, because additional factors rest within the physical environment of home and neighborhood, a third assessment is required—the *community assessment* describing possible variables that may affect the daily life of the client family.

THE FIRST ASSESSMENT: THE INDIVIDUAL

When a case referral from a physician's office arrives at a visiting nursing agency, it includes a set of orders for care. Traditionally, a nurse follows these orders to the letter and then decides that the job is complete. For community nurses, however, such a referral should present a challenge in planning care beyond just the physical measures ordered. Consequently, through the assessment, nurses should strive to get to know clients, their way of living, and their strengths and shortcomings. The assessment should include areas of health and daily living which present current or potential problems to clients. To the nurse the assessment is a blueprint for all teaching. However, the assessment is more than just a mental exercise the nurse is practicing for the sake of a care plan. Since the assessment includes all facets of life that prevent clients from fully taking advantage of their bodies and minds, it may present them with a first step from illness to well-being or from depression to happiness.

Nurses in all settings should have opportunities to engage in community health assessments, since they are the primary tool for the practice of *holistic* care. The holistic view regards the client as not only a biological being but also a psychological and sociocultural one (Pasquali, Alesi, Arnold, Debasio 2, 1981). The aim of holistic care is better physical and emotional health—something that is discussed much but practiced little in in-patient settings. In addition, Archer and Fleshman (35 and 53, 1979) believe the concept of holism in nursing often neglects environmental health, which they see as an important component of the *OLOF* (Optimum Level of Functioning) ecosystem influencing the client. Within the context of holism, then, the OLOF should be understood as being synonymous with the definition of health stated by the World Health Organization—that is, health is a state of complete physical, mental, and social well-being and not merely the absence of disease or infirmity (WHO, 1971). OLOF is an excellent concept for explaining the purpose of the community health assessment and consequent care. OLOF is achieved through holistic care. Holistic care therefore includes the three categories of prevention: *primary prevention*, in which potential problems are anticipated; *secondary prevention*, in which present problems are solved; and *tertiary prevention*, in which the damage caused by previous problems is overcome as much as possible. Let me discuss these three levels of prevention.

Primary Prevention: Prevention of Illness Through Health Promotion

Most clients are seen in medical facilities or visited by public health nurses because they have a medical problem. Few people recognize the value of seeking primary prevention care. However, community nurses who see clients during medical emergencies and win their trust are in a good position to introduce them to primary prevention. A nurse may present a client and his or her family with the option of a thorough primary-prevention assessment and, depending on the results of this assessment, several sessions of preventive teaching. Ideally, the option should not depend on the nurse's schedule or personal preference but should rest entirely with the client. The assessment and teaching plan should be discussed with the family and enthusiastically recommended if family's willingness, schedule, financial situation permit. However, if motivation is lacking, it is almost impossible for learning to take place (Smitherman,

126, 1981). Certain families may be unable to recognize the value of preventive teaching, even though the assessment shows much care is desperately needed. In such a case, the community nurse may need to make several visits in order to build trust and get the family to want to listen.

If clients do show interest in primary prevention, they need to know the content areas that the nurse plans to assess. Table 1-1 offers suggestions for a lifestyle and preventive health assessment. Though by no means complete, it encompasses the main areas of primary prevention and is geared to people without physical problems or chronic disease who nonetheless need to prevent illness through a healthy way of living. (Clients with such medical and psychological problems are discussed later in the chapter.)

To begin a primary nursing care assessment, the nurse should first present the family with an outline of the seven areas he or she plans to cover—namely:

1. Physical condition
2. Diet and fluids and elimination
3. Activity and rest patterns
4. Life enjoyment and satisfaction
5. Social support system
6. Stress and stress prevention
7. Preventive medical, dental, and eye care

The first area is assessed by means of a physical exam. The second through seventh areas are described in the accompanying table.

Second, the nurse should make a quick assessment of the client's problems and individual interests. This will allow the nurse to emphasize the areas the client perceives as important or problematic.

Next, the nurse should make the actual assessment, doing separate assessments for each family member. If time permits, a complete or partial physical assessment should be performed, if not already done in a clinic or hospital or if such records are not available. A health history should precede or follow the physical assessment, and may often be obtained from hospital or clinic records.

With these steps completed, the community health nurse is ready to interview the client about the six areas listed in Table 1-1, leading to a complete individual assessment. Sample questions will be described in Chapter 4.

TABLE 1-1 PRIMARY PREVENTION: SIX ASSESSMENT AREAS

Diet and Fluids and Elimination:

Knowledge of the four food groups and actual integration of knowledge into meal preparation
Amounts of food consumed daily from each food group
Fluids—what kinds of drinks and how many taken per day
Alcoholic beverages—what kind and how many
Snacks—what kind, how much, how often consumed
Frequency of meals
Likes and dislikes of foods
Eating habits—where, when, how fast eaten, with whom eaten
Emotional aspects with regard to eating
Patterns of elimination—frequency, constipation or diarrhea, laxatives

Activity and Rest Patterns:

Employment or regular occupation—hours, satisfaction with work
Physical activity other than work—type of activities, time involved
Sleep and rest patterns
Hobbies and activities other than sports and physical exercise—type of activities, time involved

Life Enjoyment and Satisfaction:

Maslow's needs: Level of fulfillment
Physical needs—ability to provide food, drink, clothing, shelter, sexual needs
Security needs—physical safety, emotional security, religion financial security
Need for self-esteem and esteem by others—achievements, goals, self-concept, responsibilities, authority

Social Support Systems:

Family support—members of nuclear and extended family, emotional closeness
Friendship circle—number of friends, how close, skills in making friends, aspects of life shared with friends
Social circle—participation in social activities, clubs, community activities, visiting and being visited, relationships at work, aspects of life shared with casual acquaintances
Religious support—meaning of religion, social contacts through religious institution

Stress and Stress Prevention:

Presence of stress—severity as perceived by client, frequency of high-stress incidents, emotional reactions to stress, physical symptoms related to stress
Sources of stress—for example, work situation, home and family, achievement
Coping methods—used at present, used in the past

Preventive Medical, Dental, and Eye Care:

Medical care providers—regular, emergency, specialists
Dental and eye care providers
Frequency of preventive visits
Health insurance
Birth control and VD prevention
Communicable disease prevention—immunization, TB tests, awareness of transmission, prevention, cleanliness, hygiene, food preservation

Secondary Prevention:
Needs of the Ill Client

When visiting a family, the community nurse will usually find one well-identified patient and should first direct care toward that person. However, after doing a thorough primary prevention assessment, the nurse may find that other family members have physical or emotional symptoms of illness as well which make them candidates for secondary prevention. The nurse must then decide whether the problems can be handled by nursing care or whether the client family needs a referral to another health-care provider. Such a decision can be objectively reached as the nurse collects data in more detail. Data collection centered around a client's physical or emotional problem is a secondary prevention assessment. The first part of the assessment involves the ill client who has been diagnosed by either the physician or the nurse. Table 1-2 pinpoints the assessment areas involved. (Sample questions will be described in Chapter 5.)

The areas described in Table 1-2 are specific to the ill person; however, the total secondary prevention assessment includes all areas of the primary assessment as well. The two assessments combined will provide detailed information regarding the various factors that interfere with physical and emotional well-being. However, this time the assessment of the areas mentioned under primary prevention will be more complex, since they must be looked at from two angles—the state they were in prior to illness and the state they are in at the present time.

TABLE 1-2 SECONDARY PREVENTION—PHYSICAL OR EMOTIONAL PROBLEMS: ASSESSMENT AREAS

Nursing care procedures required—ordered treatments, equipment needed, availability and condition, cleaniness

Comfort of ill client—positioning, pain, cleanliness of body and surroundings

Safety of ill client

Disease process—nature of problem, state of healing, expected symptoms, prognosis, physiological processes involved

Interference with physical functioning—client's ability to participate in treatment and daily activities, discrepancy between previous and present level of function, expected permanent loss of function

Interference with emotional well-being, discrepancy between previous and present levels

In addition, the nurse should write a statement of progress about the client. For example, in an assessment of activity and rest patterns, a nurse might note the following about employment or regular daily occupation:

Client previously worked full time, regular day shift, as sales clerk for J.C. Penney. Now unable to remain in standing position longer than 30 min at a time. Is on illness leave but sees no possibility of returning to the same job. During hospitalization she was tested by OT department for possible retraining to a sedentary job. Results pending.

Putting such detail in the assessment data helps depict the diversity of problems that are secondary to the physical problem, such as depression, sleeplessness, lack of energy, social isolation, and tension between family members.

The second part of the assessment concentrates on other family members, specifically those persons taking care of the client. Table 1-3 outlines a few areas that need to be considered by the nurse. These caretakers need to be taught caretaking procedures and made aware of the client's needs.

A primary assessment of the caretakers will be of particular value if the community nurse attempts to anticipate problems that might arise. For example, if a caretaker shows bouts of insomnia and depressive reactions every time his or her spouse is discharged from the hospital, this signals coping weaknesses, requiring extra support and reassurance by the nurse in order to stimulate the caretaker's confidence.

All the assessment areas outlined in Tables 1-1 through 1-3 are closely related and often influence each other. It is apparent that community nurses should try to understand the whole problem as it increases stress and inhibits needs from being met.

TABLE 1-3 CARETAKER ABILITY AND MOTIVATIONS: ASSESSMENT AREAS

Background and previous experience in care of ill people

Intelligence; ability to follow instructions, understand concepts

Dexterity

Commitment to ill person's care

Understanding of the nature of the client's problems

Level of coping with increased stress

Tertiary Prevention: Potential for Rehabilitation and Adjustment to Loss

A client in need of tertiary prevention is one who is suffering from damage resulting from a previous physical or mental illness condition or who is adjusting to a chronic condition and for whom the damage may gradually increase and abilities decrease. The assessment areas of tertiary prevention are the same as those in secondary prevention, with the emphasis on rehabilitation.

Whether the treatment is weightlifting, colostomy care, or recreational therapy, it is aimed at overcoming the effects of the previous disease and making the task of coping somewhat easier for the client. Such ways of coping are often overlooked unless there is a tertiary care assessment and a statement of progress made. The statement of progress describes the condition before the illness, the present condition, ways the client has coped with the changes, and contributions of family members and friends. For example, a statement of progress in the area of stress and its prevention might read as follows:

> *Previously, the client's stress was work related, mostly owing to high demand for performance and insufficient positive feedback from superiors. Stress at present is illness related, stemming from frustrations owing to immobility, and feelings of uselessness resulting from the inability to perform the work that previously provided some recognition and self-esteem.*
>
> *Stress is evidenced by the client's irritability and short temper, which affects his relationship with his wife and children. The client is not willing to participate in family activities, isolates himself, and demands to be left alone.*
>
> *BP is 140/82, elevated somewhat compared to previous levels.*
>
> *Client is coping poorly with stress and gets severely depressed and withdrawn. Previously he coped with stress by using physical outlets—playing ball, running, and swimming. He has never openly shared his feelings with wife or friends.*

The above assessment areas present a basis for nursing diagnosis and a plan for care. Other areas such as religion and culture should also be looked at by the nurse to see if the teaching approach should be modified. Religion was mentioned in Table 1-1 under the assessment areas of "Life enjoyment and satisfaction" and "Social support systems." People's spiritual needs are closely related to their needs for security, since they are striving for peace of mind in the belief in a higher force and purpose. Their sense of security comes from the assurance that they are supported in their struggles and eventually rewarded for them. People practicing religion usually do so with others; they feel part of a community in which they are accepted and respected. Therefore, religion not only helps provide a social support system but also gives them a sense of identity and a healthy self-concept.

Religion permeates many aspects of life, influencing thinking, emotional experience, behavior, and reactions to extraneous happenings, and the same holds true for culture. Certain beliefs, values, and morals, which are passed on from generation to generation, are integral parts of people's self-systems. They influence not only what kind of foods and entertainment they like but also the child development, methods of adaptation within the community, stance toward life, and self-perception. Culture may determine to what degree people are affected by stress. For example, one study shows that in the Mexican culture low education and low income do not affect a person's self-esteem, but in the White or Black culture they do (Mirowski & Ross, 1980). Thus, what is stressful or frustrating to some people is not to others, and the factor that makes the difference between the two groups is culture or values.

Religion is relatively easy to assess because people are able to tell the nurse what they believe in. However, culture has not previously been incorporated in assessments because clients are not usually aware of how cultural mechanisms affect them. Thus, culture cannot easily be assessed with an interview but must be deduced from the way a family interacts with the nurse. Even so, awareness of cultural factors is extremely important since they greatly affect the client-nurse relationship and may determine whether a family will accept nursing care or not. Teaching methods need to be adapted so they become compatible with the client's value system. Techniques for increasing awareness of cultural factors are discussed in Part III.

THE SECOND ASSESSMENT: THE FAMILY

In assessing the family, the community nurse should not be unduly concerned with the structure or nature of the family—that is, with its composition in terms of who lives with whom and for how long—lest he or she be misled by nontraditional family arrangements and fall into a net of value judgments, ignoring the actual roots of functional problems. To determine whether a family is functional, the nurse should consider a list of family functions, such as those given in Duvall, *Family Development* (114–116, 1977):

1. Generating affection
2. Providing personal security and acceptance
3. Giving satisfaction and a sense of purpose
4. Assuring continuity of companionship
5. Guaranteeing social placement and socialization
6. Inculcating controls and a sense of what is right

For practical purposes, the nurse making a family assessment needs to determine which functions are actually affected by a problem. Of course causal relationships are at times difficult to establish, since a problem will affect not just one person or aspect of family life but many. A father losing his job, for example, will first feel the effect himself, but as his role as provider is affected, it may disturb the family's security (Duvall's second function), the father's self-esteem and emotional well-being (Duvall's third function), and the family's love and affection for each other (Duvall's first function). Thus, such an event will affect every facet of that family's existence. Illness, too, can have severe consequences for family functioning.

Responses to an event such as unemployment or illness may be overwhelming for a community nurse trying to grasp what is actually going on. The question of whether a family is functional is made easier if the nurse thinks in terms of Maslow's needs, as shown in Table 1-1, "Life Enjoyment and Satisfaction" (Goble, 1971). People live together because that makes it easier for them to meet their individual needs. Ideally, they share love and affection, support each other, provide security, and help each other cope with difficulties. Family members find fulfillment and self-esteem through other members who support them, accept them, and permit them to grow physically and emotionally.

Because the family is the unit that most strongly influences its individual members' well-being, the assessment should look at how the family affects each individual member. The assessment is most effectively done by comparing the ideal (of sharing love and affection, and so on, as mentioned above) with actual circumstances. If the aim of individuals is to meet their needs to a great extent within the family, then the family can be termed functional if it serves that purpose. The community should be looked at in similar terms, complementary to the family in meeting individual needs. Changes only need to occur if neither of the two provide an environment of health and room to grow for the individual.

Since people within the family influence each other, compete with each other, make compromises, and give up some benefits for the good of another member, the task is more complex than just looking at each individual separately. Thus, the family has to be looked at as a total unit, where members function as parts. An easy way to start is to look at the physical setting of the home. The home influences many aspects of family life—communication patterns, pastime activities, and division of labor—but it also gives clues as to values the family holds—whether the family values cleanliness, art, or plants, for example. Photographs may indicate emotional ties with the extended family. Books in a shelf may point out family members' professional and diversional interests.

An assessment of the home may be done efficiently with assessment forms available in agencies, or you can construct your own (see Table 1-4).

TABLE 1-4 THE HOME: ASSESSMENT AREAS

Appearance of the house, style, type of construction

Yard and surroundings—fences, flowers, trees, size of yard, condition

Living area—size, number of rooms, carpets, furniture, decorative objects, neatness, books

Bedrooms—number, size, furnishing, cleanliness

Kitchen—size, cleanliness, appliances, equipment

Bathrooms—plumbing, adequacy, size

Other work areas—basement, sewing room, tool shop, garage, and so on

---

The appearance of the home is a reliable indicator of the lifestyle of a family, which is closely related to socioeconomic factors (see Table 1-5).

TABLE 1-5 SOCIOECONOMIC FACTORS: ASSESSMENT AREAS

Level of income of the family—type of income, health insurance

Extent of luxuries—in the house, recreation spending, private schools, number of cars, and so on

Apparent deficiencies—in the home (food, space, clothes), recreation, school, transportation

Financial problems—debts, difficulties with budgeting, expensive habits (drugs, alcohol, gambling)

Questions of the sort suggested by Tables 1-4 and 1-5 are often difficult to ask. The nurse should previously establish a satisfactory working relationship, use tact in asking questions, and give the client the option of disclosing his or her situation in detail or not (see Chapter 9).

A further area to assess is the immediate surroundings, neighborhood, school, and other facilities with which the family has frequent contact (see Table 1-6).

**TABLE 1-6 THE IMMEDIATE COMMUNITY:
ASSESSMENT AREA**

Neighborhood—type, friendliness of neighbors, safety, appearance of homes, cleanliness

School—distance, transportation, size, satisfaction with services

Recreational possibilities—playgrounds, parks nearby, transportation necessary, use by family

Shopping facility mostly used—transportation needed

Work (father and mother)—distance, transportation

Hospital or doctor's office mostly used—satisfaction, distance, emergency plan

Church—distance, how often visited

The individual assessment for each member has given the nurse the necessary information to assess how well each member meets Maslow's needs. Any shortcomings in the area are likely to point to functional problems of the total family, especially if several members in the family complain about similar problems. For example, if a husband complains that his wife does not show any affection or ignores him unless they have a full-scale fight and the wife reports that her husband spends all of his weekend at work and has stopped taking her out for dinner, the community health nurse may suspect that self-esteem based on understanding and mutual respect for each other is deficient and that the problem is family centered. As a result, the next step of the assessment should be an examination of interaction patterns and communication patterns (see Tables 1-7 and 1-8).

**TABLE 1-7 INTERACTION PATTERNS:
ASSESSMENT AREAS**

Areas of common interest of the total family

Time spent together as a family

Time spent helping each other with chores—schoolwork, cleaning, cooking

Roles assumed by family members

Division of labor

Cultural practices and rituals

TABLE 1-8 COMMUNICATION PATTERNS: ASSESSMENT AREAS

Communication between adult members—time spent in discussion, nature of subjects discussed, usual outcome of discussions

Communication between adults and children—time spent in discussion, nature of subjects discussed, usual outcome of discussions

Emotional disclosure—ability of adults to share problems and talk about feelings, ability of adults to listen to children's problems and give emotional support

Relationship between adults—love and affection component, satisfaction with relationship, number and severity of fights and arguments, resolution of arguments

Relationship between adults and children—love and affection component, reaction of children to simple commands, methods of discipline, amount and severity of discipline by either adult, reaction of child to discipline

Relationship between children—cooperative play, amount of fighting and severity, presence of concern for each other and helping each other

---

In order to get questions of this nature answered, the interviewer must be skilled in communication techniques as well as able to build a therapeutic relationship with a family. Some answers cannot be obtained by asking questions; they have to be observed. Answers need to be noted with caution, since questions such as "severity of discipline" are often not answered with perfect honesty. At times, if the problem is difficult to assess and statements of the father contradict the mother's, the nurse needs to visit the children's teacher, a doctor, a minister, or other people with whom the family has contact. If one adult blames the other, but the partner is not present to defend himself or herself, the community nurse needs to be cautious about forming judgments. In fact, to be effective, the community nurse should stay neutral, recognizing that the roots of communication problems are not as obvious as they appear, that any one part of the family system is not likely to have caused the problem independently of all the others, and that (after some in-depth probing) unmet needs will become evident in all family members.

The last area (Table 1-9), the family's health practices and attitudes toward health, is probably the most important part of the family assessment. However, the information may not be as openly available as one might think. Many attitudes are not manifested until, for example, the client is asked to have his or her eyes tested but forgets a clinic appointment three times in a row. Culture is incorporated in health attitudes. Beliefs a person's grandmother held may still be influencing that person's decisions in spite of the medical principles and the nurse's attempts to teach scientific facts.

TABLE 1-9 HEALTH PRACTICES AND ATTITUDES TOWARD HEALTH: ASSESSMENT AREAS

Frequency of use of medical services

Kind of medical services used by family

Illness prevention practiced by family—awareness of relationship diet–health, relaxation–health, exercise–health; actual practices—diet, relaxation, exercise

Self-treatment, self-medication

Self-diagnosis—temperature taking, blood pressure, weight, urine

Hygiene and cleanliness

Attitude toward pain

If the family assessment is done for the purpose of secondary or tertiary prevention, it should be handled in the same way as the individual assessment. With the problem of the ill family member kept in mind, all areas should be assessed, first as they were before the illness and then as they are at present. A statement of progress should also be prepared, indicating the coping of the family with the problem. For example, a statement of progress about Lena and her family might be as follows:

Roles assumed by family members:

1. *Lena:* Being the eldest child, the girl has previously assisted Mother with cleaning and cooking and has watched younger siblings during Mother's frequent absences. At present, Lena is confined to bed in her room. She still entertains the little boy by reading books to him and by playing games for a few hours every evening.

2. *Mother* has adapted by cutting down work hours and social visits. She complains often about this and seems unhappy.

3. *Mother's friend Melissa* helps with the morning care of Lena and goes shopping for the family.

4. *Herb (son)* cleans house on Saturdays and cooks an occasional meal. He performs these chores cheerfully.

THE THIRD ASSESSMENT: THE COMMUNITY

The community assessment is usually highly recommended and valued in textbooks but neglected by practicing community nurses. Often the community assessment is assigned to inexperienced student nurses as a learning experience. The reason why experienced community nurses do not do such assessments is because after they have been practicing for a while they feel they have "internalized" the community of which they are part, and feel they know the good and bad sections of town, the insides of tenements, the schools, the city parks and playgrounds, the medical and social services, and the major hospitals. All this knowledge seems to make community assessments useless.

Community nurses as a rule give care to individuals. Agencies are structured in such a way that even family-centered care remains a textbook ideal. Because visiting nurses need a doctor's referral to visit a patient, this automatically excludes many families who might seek care not for illness but for health promotion. In addition, the nurse's patient load is such that he or she does not have the time to do physical assessments on all family members and conduct a two-hour interview. Clinic nurses are under even more severe time pressure, being obliged to move clients through the clinic quickly so as not to waste physicians' and clients' time. To practice family care, therefore—and certainly to perform community assessments—a community nurse must either be an independent practitioner or be a firm believer in the cause of holistic nursing.

As long as individual nursing care or family nursing care is the aim of community health nursing, a detailed community assessment is not necessary. The immediate community assessment shown in Table 1-6, when performed as part of the family assessment, is adequate, for it touches the main systems the family interacts with in the community. At times, special problems will come up in an assessment—for example, a baby has elevated lead levels or a sixth-grade hiker is covered with a rash caused by poison ivy—and such problems will need to be investigated in more detail. If the baby spends more time at a daycare center and some at her grandmother's house, both sites will need to be investigated for possible sources of lead. For the sixth-grader, the nurse should find out what trails in what park the child used, so that county park employees may perhaps remove such plants. In both cases, the community nurse's reactions involve assessment of parts of the community in order to prevent further damage, and the assessments are delegated to other professionals.

Ideally, the community assessment should be done as a combined effort by all groups of people working with people and systems of people in that community. Much of these data are readily available to every community agency. The census data is broken down into local areas as small as city blocks. Census tracts are areas of approximately 4000 people with relative homogeneity with regard to socioeconomic status and other living conditions. These units are easy to work with and provide a broad picture of what the inhabitants are like. Information available through the US Census includes that shown in Table 1-10.

TABLE 1-10 INFORMATION AVAILABLE THROUGH THE US CENSUS

Population characteristics:

Age of population
Number of males and females
Number of families
Number of families headed by females
Number and ages of children per family
Marital status
Ethnic origin—languages spoken, immigration information

Income characteristics:

Range of income
Source of income
Number of people in each income category
Number of families on public assistance

Work situation:

Hours worked presently, in past year
Unemployment—seeking work
Employer and type of job
Location of work
Transportation to work

Health information:

Chronic physical or mental condition
Disability affecting work
Disability affecting use of public transportation

Other information:

Education—highest grade completed
Family living quarters—type, size, condition, utilities, heating, facilities
Property—size, value
Costs—rent, utilities, fuel, property taxes
Commodities—telephone, air-conditioning, cars, vans and trucks
Mortgage, insurance
Population mobility (where lived five years ago)
Military service

Vital statistics are easily available as well. However, they are not broken down as conveniently as those given in the census. In addition, many agencies collect their own data from client records. Publicly supported agencies are required by law to share such information with interested persons.

An extensive problem affecting comprehensive health care is the lack of interest in sharing information and unwillingness of agencies to coordinate their services. Some agencies are operated with a self-centered attitude and individual budget. In most instances, the people in such systems are knowledgeable about only a few other systems and are only willing to use them to complement their own services. As a rule, however, system boundaries are quite impermeable; for example, when a mental health agency refers clients for child counseling or family counseling, it operates by a fixed plan. The complementary services comprise only a few agencies, which are widely used by all counselors in the agency. Indeed, there may be a dozen other agencies in the community whose services may be far superior to the ones used, but the people at the agency in question may find it easier to pursue the old referral routing.

An assessment of community services (see Table 1-11) would be ideal for the purposes of rendering health service more efficient. Today all kinds of information about a community can be stored in a computer system.

TABLE 1-11 COMMUNITY SERVICES: ASSESSMENT AREAS

Health personnel—number of physicians, nurses, dentists, paramedics compared with state and US figures

General hospitals—number, location, size; services—inpatient, outpatient, diagnostic, pediatric, mental health, and so on
> population served
> costs to consumer
> insurance accepted
> accreditation

Specialized inpatient facilities—same as above

Specialized outpatient facilities—same as above

Psychiatric hospitals—same as above

Mental health clinics—same as above and qualification of health care providers

Private mental health/psychiatric practices—same as above

Private MD practices—same as above

Private OD practices—same as above

Dentists—same as above

Nursing practices—same as above

Other health practices—same as above

Social service agencies—same as above, group according to similarity of services (that is, food, clothing, housing, legal, housekeeping, child care, and so on) and according to location (for the convenience of consumers without transportation)

A central information center would be extremely helpful in collecting all available data regarding the community. If all health care agencies participated, the computer could be programmed to instruct the consumer which route to follow to get the most efficient care. This information would be based on available services, capabilities of health care workers, fees charged for the service, size of the facility, accreditation, and so on. Such a system would not only help consumers find their way in a maze of fragmented health care services, but would do much to coordinate services and to increase the awareness of what is available. The numbers of users would automatically decrease if the quality of care was not satisfactory, and agencies would have to strive for continuing improvement of their services. Service evaluation could be made part of the information system as well.

Such coordination is still a project for the future, even though beginnings have been made. At present, a community assessment is still the responsibility of individual agencies, and most agencies do not do it. A community assessment is a complex and ongoing task. It seems that community service agencies appear and disappear at an accelerated rate. From one year to the next in a metropolitan area, the Yellow Pages of the telephone book have a totally changed appearance in the social service section. Because health personnel have difficulty staying informed about what is offered in the community, they prefer to keep a minimum of stable agencies as referral sources. A community assessment should be an ongoing inquiry about changes, not only concerning new agencies, but also new or discontinued services. This means that the persons in charge of the assessment should collect and incorporate all printed material announcing new services, should go through the Yellow Pages once a year, and should call new agencies for details. Clients are also valuable sources of information. They can be asked what services they have previously used and how satisfied they were with them.

Even though a list of community health services and related agencies is an important part of the community assessment, it is not the only information needed for comprehensive care. As previously mentioned, a community health nurse will get to know the community well after working within it for several years. However, certain nurses cannot do home visits with clients or see their clients' neighborhoods. Nurses practicing in clinics and hospitals cannot include community-based factors in their nursing care if they are not aware of the environment in which their clients live. The availability of such information is important for them as well as for nurses starting new jobs or changing over to new territories.

Even the visiting nurse who is well established will find information in the community assessment which provides a broader, more comprehensive picture of the community and its inhabitants than can be perceived when doing home care.

TABLE 1-12 COMMUNITY CHARACTERISTICS: ASSESSMENT AREAS

History—how community came to be, growth factors, change over time, traditions

Topographic characteristics—rivers, hills, valleys, soil composition

Weather—temperatures, rainfall, winds, and so on

Boundaries—area enclosed

Land use—industrial, housing, recreational, farming

Government—government organizations, names of influential people at different government levels, their interests and backgrounds

Cultural facilities—art, music, library, film, museum, historical society, club, recreation, sports activities

Housing—population density and distribution, housing type (homes, apartments) and density per area, condition of housing, distribution of health facilities, distribution of cultural facilities, parks, schools, churches, and protective facilities within housing areas

Utilities—electricity, water, gas services available in different housing areas, water treatment, sewage disposal

Schools—type, location; private schools—services; universities and special schools

Public transportation—buses, trains, planes, cars, carpools, bicycles

Protective services—fire department, police department (size, adequacy of services)

Communication—newspapers, radio, TV, telephone (number of users, services provided)

Certain aspects about the community are not clearly visible or observable and have to be understood with the help of statistics, history books, maps, weather records, land-use plans, and recreation planning (see Table 1-12). The best possible place to look for historical information is the local library; however, data regarding land use, boundaries, housing, utilities, and services is available from the town, city, or county administration. Newspapers and tourist information material cover cultural happenings. Understanding of public transportation, fire and police protection can be gained by approaching the service agencies in charge.

TABLE 1-13 POPULATION CHARACTERISTICS: ASSESSMENT AREAS

Vital statistics—birth, death rates; infant, neonatal, and maternal deaths

Population number and density—present time, changes with time, mobility of population

Population distribution by age, sex, and ethnic orgin; community characteristics compared with state and US

Education level—school years completed compared with state and US figures

Income level—breakdown of income per percentage of population; mean and median income

Employment statistics—percentage employment, unemployment, type of employment; full-time, part-time, female employment; main employers in community; breakdown of occupations

---

Census information available in libraries and public agencies is the most complete source for population information (see Table 1-13). Because the US Census is completed once every 10 years at the beginning of every new decade, toward the end of the decade census information in most communities will no longer be accurate. Unfortunately, no other demographic survey will provide an equally accurate breakdown into smaller geographical areas. Agencies such as chambers of commerce, employment security commissions, and local planning commissions also work with census statistics. In addition, they make information available on development trends and projection statistics, which can be used by the community nurse for a better understanding of population dynamics.

TABLE 1-14 HEALTH AND ILLNESS PATTERNS: ASSESSMENT AREAS

Leading causes of death—numbers and rates

Causes for infant, neonatal, and maternal deaths—numbers and rates

Incidence and prevalence of communicable diseases

Incidence and prevalence of chronic disease

Incidence and prevalence of other health problems—for example, substance abuse, violence (child abuse, spouse abuse, rape), accidents (traffic and others)

For health and illness patterns (see Table 1-14), the US and state departments of public health provide demographic material based on the National Health Survey, which is carried out on a continuing basis. The National Center of Health Statistics (NCHS) is the main compiler of health information on the national level; Health Systems Agencies (HSA) collect local data and are thus the main providers of data for the NCHS. Other sources the community nurse may use are insurance companies—especially Metropolitan Life, which publishes the *Statistical Bulletin*—and private agencies, such as the American Heart Association and the American Cancer Society (Archer & Fleshman, 43–45, 1979).

TABLE 1-15 ENVIRONMENTAL INFLUENCES ON HEALTH: ASSESSMENT AREAS

Causes of air pollution—traffic density, laws regarding car-exhaust regulation; industry—level of ashes, soot, irritants in air; danger of radioactive pollution—power plants, military testing; industrial hazards—asbestos, silicon, lead, mercury, and so on

Causes of water pollution—industrial wastes, sewage problems, oil spills, agricultural chemicals

Treatment of water—adequacy of filtration plants and the like; chlorination, fluoridation

Treatment of sewage—sludge process or stabilization ponds, adequacy, distance from water sources

Causes of soil pollution—solid waste disposal method, distance from living area and water source, recycling facilties

Causes of noise pollution—industry, airport traffic

Industrial hazard protection—air and water control, ventilation, safety measures, educational and medical services provided by main industrial employers

Environmental surveillance—monitoring water sources, air, industrial environment, food supply, sanitation in restaurants, public restrooms, schools

For environmental influences on health (see Table 1-15), the local branch of the US Environmental Protection Agency may be the best source of statistics and monitoring information. The sanitation department of the local health department as a rule is in charge of monitoring water sources and food as well as sanitation in restaurants and schools. The local department of social services is involved in control of sanitary standards in nursery schools and child-care centers. Information regarding sanitation in schools is available through the public school administration and the health department.

In summary, the community assessment is a working tool for all people involved in giving community care. The assessment procedure should be a joint effort: nurses of each agency should together assess the community according to their needs. The areas previously outlined help to structure such an assessment and include factors essential for nursing care.

The purpose of the community assessment is to provide broader understanding of the changes a community undergoes and of the kind of life the clients are leading, its quality and its problems. The importance of such an assessment can be appreciated only if the nurse thinks in terms of family systems interacting with and being greatly influenced by the community, its environmental and political forces, and the enormous rate of change occurring in today's society.

The community nurse needs to be familiar with the community as it presently exists and to stay current by continually updating the community assessment. A computer is extremely helpful, since it can store vast amounts of information and can make needed data quickly available to each nurse. However, since such help is not yet available for most agencies and little data sharing is done between different health care systems, the community nurses themselves must be responsible for collecting as much data as possible in order to make full use of community resources and provide the best possible care to the client.

To go about data collection, nurses working for an agency should develop an assessment form that includes the assessment areas mentioned, collects useful data, and helps in their understanding of their particular community or city neighborhood. An example of such a comprehensive assessment form is found in Tinkham and Voorhies, *Community Health Nursing* (277–290, 1977).

ASSESSMENT PROCEDURE

Considering the extensive detail needed to arrive at a complete assessment in order for the nurse to have a thorough understanding of client, family, and community, the community nurse may naturally respond by asking the question, "When does anyone have the *time* to do such an assessment?" The question is justified. Such an assessment only makes sense if it can be used and applied. The nurse has to have time to get involved with the family. If the involvement is limited to one visit only, it would be foolish to spend the time doing an assessment, which would be nothing more than an intellectual exercise.

To keep the assessment in pace with reality, the community nurse should make its length and detail dependent on:

- The availability of time for intervention
- The interest of the family in learning and making changes

- The support of the agency and the client's doctor or referring agency

Since primary prevention carries much weight in the assessment as well as in the implementation of care, a full assessment is warranted independent of the severity of the client's medical or emotional condition.

Under less than optimal conditions, the nurse should pick out the areas that are most relevant. This judgment would be based on the nurse's previous observations, possibly based on talks with and visits with the client in his or her home. Often it helps to listen to clients outline problem areas. Although they may not have a clear picture of many problems affecting their health, if the nurse concentrates on areas of interest to clients, it will ensure greater cooperation. For example, a woman may wish to get help for an obesity problem, and want the nurse to help set up a reasonable reducing diet and suggest a routine compatible with her lifestyle. The client may believe her problem is relatively simple and not require much assessment or teaching time. The community nurse can avoid the client's immediate refusal to get involved by using the diet assessment as a start and gradually adding further assessment later. If the client sees actual change coming about owing to her choice of foods, she may be willing to go on to other areas such as lifestyle and exercise.

The assessment procedure, then, varies from family to family and from client to client. However, prior to the first session the community health nurse should collect as much information as possible about the family to avoid having to ask the family questions they may have already answered more than once for other health professionals. This will also permit the nurse to spend more time with other aspects of the assessment.

Data about the family can be found in hospital and clinic records, in discussions with the family's physician, or in talking with nurses of the hospital or clinic that treated family members. (The process may, however, have to be restricted owing to legal implications regarding permission to release medical information.) Meetings with an ill family member in the hospital may also provide the nurse who will do visits in their home with clues as to family and neighborhood characteristics and special concerns.

Prior to the first visit, if the nurse is not familiar with the community, a community assessment should be done, although the assessment need not be as formal and detailed as previously described. Driving through the area to be visited will yield basic information on the area's residents, housing, schools, recreation areas, and the like. The nurse should also evaluate the area for his or her own safety. The condition of the dwellings, cleanliness of the streets and sidewalks, and the type of people seen in the street will indicate whether it is safe for the nurse to visit the family alone or whether a companion might be advisable. (Safety factors are discussed in Chapter 7.)

Having collected data previously will ease the nurse's assessment task during sessions with the family; however, the entire assessment can seldom be accomplished during just one family visit. Usually three or four are required. Family interactions, emotional well-being, and other information need to be gathered over time. A client who is depressed on one occasion, for instance, may feel better during the next visit.

The nurse who simply sits during the four visits with pad and pencil, jotting what clients report, without interpreting the data, risks making clients uncomfortable. Why all these questions? a client may ask. Why this probing in my private life? What will I get out of this? Some questions may even make clients angry and unwilling to cooperate. Thus, the assessment must not be an inquisition but an interpersonal exchange that creates a relationship of trust between the nurse and the family members. In addition, during the assessment, some important questions that are easy to answer should be taken care of, and hope should be instilled that more difficult questions may be worked out later.

Often the most efficient way of going through the assessment process is for the nurse to assess every area separately, then follow the assessment with teaching within that area before continuing to the next area. This method works well for preventive teaching. However, if problems arise, they must be examined in the context of all other areas as well, and the nurse should proceed with the total assessment before doing any further specialized teaching.

At no time can the assessment be considered complete, for changes occur continuously. During the teaching process, the nurse should continue the assessment, watching for dynamics that have not previously surfaced or for increased client intimacy and trust. Thus, it is actually impossible to keep the assessment separate from implementation or evaluation; all happen simultaneously and the format of care should allow all three to happen. The assessment form should provide space for additional information collected at a later date. If the nursing care continues over time, the total assessment should be updated and rewritten at regular intervals, particularly if more than one nurse is involved with the family. Again, a computer is handy for adding or deleting lines in an assessment file and for producing updated printouts when needed.

The intervals between overhauls of an assessment depend not only on the rate of change in assessment areas, complexity of family problems, and number of people involved within the family, but also on the office time the nurse has available in which to do the planning. The planning time spent in the office or nurses' station is necessary, however, and should not be considered a period of burdensome paperwork that removes the nurse from the bedside or home visits. Nursing care is no longer a routine task but must be carefully planned and evaluated. While this takes time, it is also a continuous learning experience for both patient and nurse. Only through conscientious planning will there be visible results based on the nurse's care rather than on pure chance. That is where the thrill and excitement enters, as the nurse discovers a healing power never encountered before—one based not only on intuition, but on rational thinking, knowledge, and planning.

EXAMPLE OF AN ASSESSMENT: THE CASE OF ROBERT FOX

Referral: Robert Fox, 55-year-old male. Retarded. Lives with 92-year-old mother.

Problem: Diabetes. Urines running 3 + and 4 +. Insulin dose had been increased two times within last month.

Doctor's order: Diabetic teaching and supervision of regime. Help with AM insulin injection. NPH insulin 12 units (1.2 cc/U 100) bid 30 min before breakfast and supper. Urine testing 9 AM.

Community Characteristics

The town is a small settlement of some 3000 inhabitants. Only about 600 of these live in the town proper, working in businesses, stores, restaurants, or nearby industry. Most people, however, live on farms in the surrounding areas. The town is in the process of growth, as some areas on its outskirts have been converted from farmland into new settlement areas where a considerable number of new homes and townhouses are under construction.

The industry of the area consists of a screw and a sheet-metal factory, as well as a lumberyard and a grist mill. In addition, there are many smaller business enterprises, such as construction and excavating companies or trucking firms.

The downtown area is quite picturesque. A river and a bridge leading across form the end of Main Street and the business area. The part of the river flowing through town is deep, and the water is still, after plunging down a little waterfall some 500 ft upstream. People use the bridge and the county park, which lies between the bridge and the waterfall, for fishing. The park has picnic tables and a playground for children.

The downtown area consists of old brick structures, the first floors of which are occupied by small businesses, stores, restaurants, two bars, a real estate office, a mortuary, and the fire department. The upstairs apartments of these buildings are rented out. The renters, most of them elderly, have been living in these apartments for a long time, some of them all their lives. The people know each other, visit each other, and share the day's happenings.

The other end of Main Street leads to an intersection and two main traffic veins proceeding up the hill into an area of old homes, two schools, and several churches. Adjacent to the intersection are the town hall on one side of the street and the old library on the other. The police department follows the library some 50 ft up on the same street.

The town government is composed of the most influential people in town. Most of them are in their fifties, and their attitudes are conservative. Except for one woman, the governing body is all male. These people express pride that the town's youth is better than the youth of surrounding larger communities—less into drugs, with fewer school dropouts, and most become good workers once they are out of school. Looking at statistics, it can easily be seen that the difference is not great and is getting smaller as the population increases in size.

The main public attractions of the town are the bars, sports events of the schools, and one movie theatre. The American Legion enjoys popularity with regularly scheduled social events. The library is used by women and children more than by men. The ceramics shop offers a series of classes, which are well attended by women and young people. Once a year the town has a small street fair at which merchants sell goods and demonstrate crafts. Other activities include a fishing derby and amusement rides for the young.

The town has four schools. Most of the students are bused to school, owing to the considerable distances. One elementary school, the original old town school, is in town along the hillside leading up from Main Street. The other three schools are built in a large complex at the south end of town, within walking distance from the oldest housing area in town, which is occupied by predominantly elderly people.

The client's housing area was built some 30 years ago and lies adjacent to the older area, stretching further up the hill, about two miles in distance from the river. The homes are one-family homes, wooden-frame structures, each with its small front and back yards. Many of the inhabitants take great pride in their yards, and the flowers and shrubs are a wholesome sight for the visitor. Two churches, a Catholic and a Methodist church, are part of the neighborhood and have served its needs ever since its existence.

The town has no medical inpatient facility. There are three local doctors, one osteopath, who has the largest practice, and two MD internists, both having their offices in town. In addition, there are several dentists, one of them being an orthodontist; a chiropractor; and a podiatrist. The County Community Mental Health Agency runs a weekly activity group in one of the churches for a small number of chronically mentally ill people maintained in families and for other individuals with adjustment problems. For all other medical and social services, the town people have to travel 15 miles east to the next city. There they find two major hospitals, numerous clinics, and mental health and social agencies. Public transportation is nonexistent in the community, with the exception of two or three taxicabs. Town people are dependent on their cars.

Besides the downtown area, the town has two shopping malls—one on the south side of town and one east—as well as an old country store in the rural area north of the town. Both malls consist of grocery stores and drugstores; one also has a hardware store. In-town shopping facilities are very limited, and most people take care of their need for clothes, equipment, and furnishings elsewhere.

Fire and police protection seem adequate. The crime rate is low. The fire department gets help from surrounding communities in case of emergencies. The town has a local newspaper but has neither a radio nor a TV station.

Population Characteristics

Vital statistics present an unclear picture, since the town people as a rule are not born in town but in nearby hospitals, and many do not die in town. Very few neonatal deaths occur in town but instead take place in hospitals in other communities.

The population is not evenly spread. Density is greater in the very small downtown area and in the settlements on the outskirts. Moderate-density housing areas with one-family homes account for most of the town's population. The rural outskirts show very low density.

The town's male/female ratio is 1.3. There is equal distribution by sex in the outer sectors of town, whereas in the inner, old areas the elderly population is predominantly female. The town people are almost exclusively of German ethnic origin. Compared with state and US population, the town people are older, have a higher rate of females, and show much less ethnic variation. Age distribution shows that 30% of the population falls within 0 to 18 years, 48% between 19 and 65, and 22% are 65 +.

Educational level is average for the county, 43% having less than high school graduation, 23% having high school education only, and 34% having at least some college education.

Median income was $15,000 for 1982. About 28% of the families had less than $10,000 per year; 6% of the population is below poverty level. Unemployment rate for 1982 is 10%, which is lower than figures for the state. The work force consists of 32% of the population. The majority of jobs are blue-collar and service jobs. Of the female population, roughly one third is gainfully employed, slightly more than half of these women work part time.

Health and Illness Patterns

Illness patterns are not accessible, since available figures of disease incidence are not broken down to local level. However, town doctors state that, to their knowledge, the town shows no unusual disease patterns. They suspect that they follow the county rates fairly closely.

Environmental Factors

The town does not have any apparent environmental health problem. Air pollution is not severe, since the two main industrial complexes are moderate in size and their capacity to pollute the air is minimal. Traffic through the town is light except at times of special events locally or in the neighboring towns. Pollution of the river or ground water has not been a major problem. The surrounding area maintains nonpolluting electronic and precision industry rather than heavy industry. Since the increase in growth has been only recent (within the last five years), space has been no problem. Sewage treatment stabilization ponds are removed from the town, and the garbage dump lies at a safe distance as well. There is a sewer system for the immediate town area and the outer housing developments. Other homes have to follow strict regulation with regard to septic tanks. Pollution in general has never been a major issue for this town. Due to the heavy use of agricultural fertilizer and pesticides, it may be advisable, however, to monitor wells and other sources of drinking water more than once every year.

Individual Assessment

Client: Robert Fox

History.   Robert is the youngest of three children. He was born three weeks premature but seemed in good health. Developmental problems showed up around age two. His speech was delayed and his gross motor development was rather slow. He walked at age 20 months. He was fearful about using the stairs, climbing, or jumping. At age three his vocabulary was minimal, and only his mother was able to understand his articulation. In kindergarten his learning disability as well as gross motor retardation was clearly detectable. Since there was no special school in the area, Robert was funnelled through the regular school system. He eventually learned elementary math skills and very basic reading. Once released from school, he did not carry a job. Due to a remaining speech impediment and recurrent anger outbreaks, he was considered unemployable.

The onset of his diabetes was at age 16. His mother has kept his medical regime under strict control; actually, there were few aspects of his life which escaped regulation and control imposed by his mother.

Some two years ago, with the mother in failing health and suffering diminishing eyesight, Mrs. Fox found diabetic care for her son increasingly difficult. Robert has taken advantage of this situation by becoming more independent, taking walks through town and cultivating his number one hobby—eating snacks and enjoying some drinks at a bar.

Physical and Mental Status Assessment Findings.   White male, 55 years old. Height: 5'8". Weight: 185 lb.

Appears obese, with protruding abdomen and plump face. Dressed in shirt and trousers. Clean hair, but somewhat disheveled and oily. Teeth straight and intact, yellow tinge, as observed without close inspection. Does not wear glasses. Eyes slightly bloodshot. Appearance of body rather plump, posture somewhat slumped; movements sluggish, gait wobbly, with feet positioned unusually far apart. No eye contact when talked to. Answers with one word to direct questions. Tone of voice raised as if angry and irritated.

Thinking seems coherent. Is oriented to time and space. Use of vocabulary hard to assess, owing to his noncommunicative manner.

Unusual physical findings: Perceives needle prick on feet—sole and arches—as slight, dull pressure. Sensation of legs normal.

Assessment of Diet and Fluids

Four Food Groups.   Concept of four food groups unknown to client. Knows that he should not eat sweets or drink alcohol. Does not understand the relationship between alcohol or food other than sweets and diabetes. Diabetes means too much sugar and that is why one does not eat sweets—this is his understanding.

Kinds and Amounts of Food and Drinks, Alcoholic Drinks.   Robert is unconcerned about meal preparation. He eats everything his mother offers him. The amount of food he consumes is hard to assess, since Mrs. Fox's memory is failing as far as regular meals go. In addition, Robert takes an afternoon and an evening walk to town, spends his pocket money on snacks and drinks, and visits a bar. If Mrs. Fox's food preparation used to be along diabetic diet rules, it is no longer so. Owing to her failing health, her daughter as well as neighbors and friends supply them with food and keep the refrigerator stocked with easy-to-prepare food such as canned spaghetti or TV dinners. Mrs. Fox still takes the preparation of breakfast seriously; she offers Robert two fried eggs and two strips of bacon on buttered toast, a glass of orange juice, and a large cup of coffee. Lunch is brought in or prepared by the daughter, and dinner consists of whatever is available.

Snacks.   Getting an accurate account of Robert's snacking habits is not possible. Robert is not communicative. He avoids answering direct questions and denies eating anything when going out. Stories about his behavior and habits are offered to the community nurse not by Robert himself but by villagers who see him in the bakery or the bar. He also snacks when watching TV—popcorn, according to Mrs. Fox.

Frequency of Meals.   Three meals are offered in the home. Snacks are consumed outside. Frequency unknown.

Likes and Dislikes of Food.   Robert does not complain about foods offered to him in the home. He eats everything he can get but has a special liking for sweet foods.

Eating Habits.   Robert eats fast. He does not want to sit down at the table for long. He seems to want to avoid socialization by devouring his food and leaving the kitchen as soon as possible. At home he eats in the kitchen, and in the living room when watching TV. He has been seen eating when walking along the street, in the bakery, and the coffee shop in town. The kitchen personnel in the American Legion offer him leftovers from dinner preparation for guests.

Emotional Aspects.   Most people Robert associates with offer him food or have drinks with him. Food is a symbol of friendship for him. It means to him that people accept and like him. Robert's obesity is a result of his attitude, and his resistance to change is great.

Assessment of Activity and Rest Pattern

Employment.   For the last two years Robert has not been working. In the past he has earned pocket money by helping to load and unload merchandise in a trucking company owned by a family friend. People there have tolerated occasional anger outbreaks and let him help whenever he felt like it, not pushing a strict time schedule. At present he is unable to continue this work, owing to weakness in his legs based on diabetic neuropathy.

Physical Activity.   His only exercise at present is the daily walks to town, 1½ miles each way. This is reflected by a weight gain of 20 lb over the last year.

Sleep and Rest Patterns.   Robert sleeps some 12 hours per day. He tends to watch TV until late or socialize with friends in the bar. His mother has difficulty getting him up in the morning for his insulin and breakfast. He gets up at 10 AM for breakfast and then goes back to bed until 12:30 to 1:00 PM.

Other Activities and Hobbies.   Robert constructs model airplanes. He is able to understand directions and follows them. He has made some planes with motors, and on sunny afternoons he flies his planes in the county park. He has also assembled racing cars. His workmanship is not perfect, but his understanding of mechanics is excellent. The home has a large basement and Robert spends most of his time there. There is a wood shop with a modern set of tools and a large workbench.

Another hobby is playing drums. Robert has at one time played with a local band and has performed for special events in town. This was more than 10 years ago, however, and at present he no longer uses the drums.

Assessment of Life Enjoyment and Satisfaction

Physical Needs.   There is no problem regarding the ability to procure food and clothing. The home is old but adequate and in good condition. Robert's sexuality at the present time does not present a problem. There are stories about him following some girls around in the past. Robert was then treated as the village fool and people laughed at his sexual approaches, which were clumsy and unskilled. Robert seems to have ceased to be interested in women. He does not offer any information on the subject.

Security Needs.   Physical safety in the home is satisfactory. Robert handles his tools with skill and has not had any accidents in the past. His noncompliance with regard to his diet poses the greatest threat to his physical health. Robert's religious conviction is hard to assess. He does not go to church, since people used to make fun of him, and he refuses to respond to questions in this area. Financial security is insured by social security checks and the support of the extended family.

Self-Esteem.   Robert gains his self-esteem by excelling at model construction. He has been able to help some neighbor boys with their models. He shows his work area with pride to anyone interested and explains in detail what he is doing. This is in great contrast to his usual grumpiness and unwillingness to communicate.

Robert also gains self-esteem by interacting with a group of town people among whom he feels accepted. He is known by everyone in town and enjoys a certain reputation. People smile at him and greet him. His being different is accepted among the adult population. There are regular incidences where children tease him and make fun of him. Robert has learned to ignore them to a great extent. He is skilled at closing up and withdrawing as soon as he hears or sees something that threatens his integrity. The community nurse has difficulties "getting through to him" since he is generally well defended and unapproachable to people he does not trust.

His self-concept is not easy to assess. He makes no derogatory remarks about himself. However, he is often withdrawn and uncommunicative. His depression is lifted by angry outbreaks, usually directed toward authority figures. His mother stated in tears that he was becoming more and more stubborn and nasty to her. His rebellion toward authority is also evidenced by his noncompliance and daily outings against advice and his refusal to get up in the morning.

He does not seem to have any goals. His dream used to be to become a well-known drum player. At present, he expresses disillusionment and disappointment that his dream did not become reality. Robert does not have any responsibility in the household or toward his mother.

Assessment of the Social Support System

The Family.   The family has strong emotional ties. The daughter, married and living close by, is the eldest in the family and takes care of mother and Robert. Robert is liked by his family, even though he gives them a hard time. Robert's older brother visits often. He has marital difficulties and he spends many nights at the family's house rather than in his own home. Mother makes him feel welcome, prepares him food, and washes his laundry. At present she is having difficulties doing this, and the daughter is taking over.

Friends and Social Circle.   Robert has a large social-support system, with many friends who like him and accept him. He is skilled in sorting out people who like him and people who do not. He does consciously seek contact with "his kind of people." Even though he isolates himself at home, among his friends he is a different person, outgoing and funny at times. His socialization pattern is quite superficial. He does a lot of listening to what others have to say and makes a remark now and then, a comment or a joke. There seems to be a sense of admiration of his friends, which probably leads them to liking him and responding in a positive manner.

Robert's best friend is his brother, whom he admires and adores. He is the only person Robert listens to. If his brother lets Robert accompany him to the bar, Robert's facial expression lights up with pride. Robert's brother is an alcoholic.

Assessment of Stress

Stress.   Robert's lifestyle does not present stress. He passes his day as he pleases, without pressures and responsibilities. Stress experienced by Robert is of intrapsychic nature—that is, stress due to frustration, which is based on deterioration of his health, his authority conflict, and his lack of physical and emotional outlets. Reactions to stress are anger, rebellion, and noncompliance. He copes by getting out of the house and associating with people who do not order him around. Coping is nonproductive, since it threatens his physical health.

Assessment of Preventive Medical, Dental, and Eye Care

Medical Care.   Robert sees the osteopathic physician, who has his practice in the house adjacent to his own, on a regular basis. The doctor has done excellent service to the community. His practice is large. He acts like a father figure for the family and helps and directs them in any kind of emergency. He has a special liking for the Fox family and suggests whatever measures they should be taking to improve their general health. He tests Robert's blood sugar on a regular basis and has alerted the family members as to the importance of diabetic diet. He has previously sent in a public health nurse to do diabetic teaching. At this point he feels that the diabetic regime is out of control and suggests that other factors be looked at and explored in order to explain Robert's noncompliance. The doctor is aware of Robert's outings as well, since news travels fast in this community. Robert has been hospitalized several times in the past for his diabetes. Tests have been done regarding the neuropathy on his legs, since Robert complains of much pain. He is angry at the doctor, since he could not make his leg pain go away.

Dental Care.   Robert's teeth are in fair condition. The mother has been sending him to a dentist on a yearly basis. Recently, however, this has not been reinforced, and even though the medical doctor has advised him to see a dentist, Robert refused to make an appointment. His teeth are in need of repair, since his dental hygiene is rather poor.

Eye Care.   Robert's eyesight has deteriorated in the last year or two. He has difficulty reading instructions on his model sets. He refuses to follow his doctor's advice about seeing an eye doctor.

Preventive Visits.   Robert does not see the doctor for other reasons than his diabetic checkups or for emergencies. The doctor gives him a physical exam once a year and reassesses his health status regularly.

Communicable Disease Prevention.   Robert had the usual childhood diseases early in life. His regular TB tests are negative. Robert's practices of hygiene and cleanliness seem satisfactory; however, his mother keeps reminding him of showers and complains that it becomes more and more troublesome, as Robert is not very cooperative.

The family has a functioning refrigerator. However, some foods are left on the table for several hours after meals before Mrs. Fox remembers to put them back into the refrigerator.

Assessment for Secondary Prevention

The Problem.   Diabetes since age 16. Presently poorly controlled. Daily urine tests running 3 + and 4 +. Neuropathy of legs. Possible diabetic retinopathy.

Pain.   Robert complains of pain in thighs and calves, especially upon getting up in the morning. Failing strength prevents him from doing work involving heavy lifting. The pain itself does not seem incapacitating at present.

Progression.   The condition has taken a turn for the worse, especially during the last two years. Possibly it can be halted by better compliance with a medical regime.

Interference.   Robert seems to react emotionally to the deterioration. He shows more anger and depression.

Treatment.   This consists of the usual diabetic regime—diet 1500 cal and insulin; see the doctor's order. Urine testing is required daily in the morning. Hygiene, especially foot care, is required. Regular physical exercise is necessary.

Equipment.   The family purchases insulin and syringes. Insulin is kept in the refrigerator. They also purchased a urine testing kit.

Treatment Procedure.   Diet: See primary care assessment. Injections: Not done by client. The client's sister comes in all evenings, weekend mornings, and two other mornings. On three mornings, the mother takes over with much difficulty, since she cannot see well. The client's sister draws up the insulin on the previous evening. Robert's sister complains that the responsibility is getting to be too much for her. Robert is supposed to do his own urine tests, but forgets often.

Assessment for Tertiary Prevention

The Problem.   Progression of diabetes has influenced Robert's ability to pursue his daily activities and his emotional well-being.

Treatment.   Comprehensive evaluation is needed of Robert's abilities in order to help him adjust current activities to his physical restrictions or introduce new activities geared to his intellectual and physical capacity.

Treatment Procedure.   Use community resources.

Individual Assessment

Client.   Edna Fox

History.   Mrs. Fox has enjoyed extremely good physical health all her life. She had three children without complications. Widowed at age 47, she independently completed the job of raising her children, and earned money cleaning houses and doing ironing for other people. Her health started to fail about six months ago. She states that she just does not feel good anymore, is tired all the time, and has no energy. She has become forgetful and unable to manage her household efficiently, a fact that bothers her greatly. She saw the doctor for a cold she could not get rid of and was then found to have high blood pressure. The doctor prescribed medication, but ever since she started taking it she complained she has not felt like herself, so she stopped taking it.

Physical and Mental Status Assessment Findings.   White female, 92 years old. Height: 5'1". Weight: 92 lb.

Mrs. Fox appears thin and fragile. Her facial expression is tired and weary, but her eyes are alert and inquisitive. She is usually dressed in a grey cotton dress, clean and tidy. Her hair is rather thin and white, tied in a knot. She has dental prostheses, two full plates. Her body posture is erect. Her gait is slow but coordinated. She has good eye contact, is talkative, and seems to enjoy sharing problems. Her voice is moderate in volume, and her hearing is good. Her emotional affect is normal, her general mood sad and discouraged. Her thinking pattern is productive, but she has difficulties remembering details that happened in the recent past.

Unusual physical findings: BP 168/106. Weakness in left arm and hand—difficulties squeezing nurse's hand and doing straight arm lift with a cup in her hand. Right arm normal. Eyesight poor. Wears reading glasses. Cataracts diagnosed by MD.

Assessment of Diet and Fluids

Four Food Groups.   Mrs. Fox has never heard about the four food groups, but she has a fairly good understanding as to what should be included in a balanced diet. She has a basic understanding of a diabetic diet. She has some difficulties working with exchanges, especially with regard to size of portions. In the past she has served sample menus rather than substituted one food for another. She realizes that Robert is not complying with his diet and worries about it. She does not keep sugar or honey in the house.

Kinds and Amounts of Foods, Drinks, and Alcoholic Beverages.
Mrs. Fox states that she is "just not hungry anymore." She eats an egg
and toast for breakfast, and some soup or a few bites of whatever there is
in the refrigerator for dinner. Lunch is brought in by the daughter. She is
taking vitamin pills the doctor prescribed for her, since she cannot chew
most fresh food and does not feel like having vegetables often. She likes
a glass of red wine before bedtime. She drinks two cups of coffee and about
two glasses of water per day. She dislikes milk.

Snacks. None.

Frequency of Meals. Regular three meals, supper being very small.

Likes and Dislikes. Mrs. Fox has lost her taste for vegetables and
her interest in foods in general, saying "they all taste the same." She used
to like fresh fruit but has trouble chewing. She gets most enjoyment from
her two cups of coffee in the morning and the evening. She refuses milk
but eats milk products. She likes bread, especially homemade bread.

Eating Habits. She eats regularly, usually with Robert in the kitchen.
During that time she attempts to communicate with him, since he usually
hides in the basement. She eats slowly.

Emotional Aspects. Food does not mean anything to her anymore.
Possible loss of taste.

Assessment of Activity and Rest Pattern

Daily Activities. Mrs. Fox used to take great pride in her house and
garden. Only six months ago she had still done a great deal of her cleaning,
washing, and cooking and some vegetable gardening. At present she prepares breakfast. If her daughter does not stay for dinner, she will serve
some fast foods. She still washes the laundry and does some dusting, but
heavier cleaning has become too much for her.

The work in the house is her only activity. She does not go out of the
house anymore, except when her daughter takes her to town.

Sleep and Rest Patterns. Mrs. Fox has slept eight hours per day for
many years. She had a strict routine, with a regular bedtime, and she
would wake up fresh and energetic. During the last year her sleep has been
lighter. She has many "bad dreams" and she wakes up two to three times
during the night. In the morning she feels tired. She forces herself to do
her routine, but after lunch she needs to lie down for another nap. Even

though she spends more time in bed, she does not seem to get the same amount and quality of sleep she got before.

Other Activities.   Mrs. Fox used to take great pride in her garden as well as in cooking, and visited with friends. These hobbies became too much of an effort for her during the last year. She gave up her regular walk to town two years ago. Until recently she still took smaller walks in the neighborhood. At present she lacks the energy.

Assessment of Life Enjoyment and Satisfaction

Physical Needs.   (See Robert Fox.) Mrs. Fox has been "faithful to her husband and never loved anyone else" since his death at age 47.

Security.   Up to this point Mrs. Fox has been managing independent living satisfactorily. Her failing memory is a potential danger. So far there have been no incidents of forgetting to turn off the stove and the like. She has not had any falls and walks stairs well. Her balance is good. Her failing eyesight also is potentially dangerous.

Self-Esteem.   Mrs. Fox used to derive her self-esteem from being independent and managing her household as well as from taking care of her children. At present she is depressed as a result of her failing health. Another factor influencing her depression is the feeling that she has lost control over Robert. In the past her responsibility for taking care of Robert seems to have kept her young and active. Now she knows that she is failing and so is Robert. This is a great worry. No arrangements have been made as to what would happen to Robert when she dies.

Social Support System.   (See Robert Fox.) The most helpful people are daughter and the doctor. Neighbors are very concerned and come to visit regularly.

Assessment of Stress

Stress.   Stress is based on the factors outlined under "Self-Esteem."

Assessment of Preventive Medical, Dental, and Eye Care

Medical Care.   Mrs. Fox has had regular physical examinations, because her doctor has reminded her of them when she has brought Robert in for tests. Lately she has been in the doctor's office frequently. She has tried several medications he prescribed and did not like their side effects. She stated that she goes to see the doctor whenever she feels bad enough.

Dental Care.   Mrs. Fox has not seen a dentist since her plates were made.

Eye Care.   An eye doctor was seen about a year ago. At that point Mrs. Fox was told that she had cataracts but that they had not progressed enough for eye surgery. She has glasses for reading but states that they do not do much good.

Communicable Disease Prevention.   Mrs. Fox is very conscious of personal hygiene and cleanliness. She takes daily showers in a walk-in shower. There is a handlebar to hold for safety.

Regular TB tests are negative.

Food practices: See Robert Fox.

Assessment for Secondary and Tertiary Prevention

The Problem.   Old age, high blood pressure probably due to arteriosclerotic disease. Stress factor may be involved. Weakening heart muscle.

Pain.   None.

Progression.   See primary prevention assessment.

Interference.   See primary prevention assessment.

Treatment.   None except for vitamins. She has a prescription for digitoxin 0.1 mg daily and Aldactazide 1 tablet bid. She has complained of weakness, light-headedness, and just "not being herself" when taking the pills.

Family Assessment: The Home

Appearance.   The home is about 30 years old, a white, wood-frame structure. There are five steps leading up to the front porch. The covered wooden porch is large enough for a small table and two to three lawn chairs. There is a back door leading into the kitchen. Some 10 flower pots and herb plants are kept outside the back door. The outside of the house is in good condition; there are no broken windows, and the house has been repainted recently.

Yard. There is a yard with a small lawn and flower beds around it, mostly perennial shrubs. Several big trees, pines, are in the back and a large ash tree is in front.

Living Area. The one-story home has three bedrooms, a bathroom, a living room, a small kitchen, and a full basement. The living room has a grey carpet and is furnished with a couch, coffee table, and two armchairs, as well as an antique buffet with a bookshelf. Several plants decorate the room along the two windows, some on the sills, some hanging from the ceiling. Wall hangings consist of one painting—a present of a hobby-painter friend, Mrs. Fox said—and family photographs. Small framed photographs are also exhibited on the buffet and the large TV set. Colors in the living room are subdued—grey, brown, and beige curtains.

Bedrooms. The bedrooms are used by Robert and Mrs. Fox, and the third one by Mrs. Fox's older son, who sleeps over quite often. Robert's room is cluttered with stacks of papers, a pile of laundry on a chair, and model planes and cars on the dresser and on the floor. It is very small, just enough room for the bed, a dresser, and a chair. Mrs. Fox's room is larger. Its furnishings consist of a double bed, two chests of drawers, a little dresser with mirror, a chair, and two nightstands. Photographs decorate her room as well, some of them of her husband. The third room appears much like Robert's except that, instead of being cluttered with models, it has stacks of magazines, such as news magazines, sex magazines, and detective stories.

Bathroom. The bathroom is small, with a walk-in shower, sink, and toilet. The plumbing is functioning and, except for an agglomeration of toiletry bottles on the shelf above the sink and on the water tank behind the toilet, it looks neat and clean.

Kitchen. The kitchen is very small, and many utensils, pots, and pans have to be kept on the counter, owing to lack of storage space. The breakfast dishes piled in the sink and the greasy frying pan on the kitchen table give it a cluttered, untidy appearance. The refrigerator is in working order but is in need of cleaning. Cooking is done with electricity. The kitchen table and four chairs are used extensively by the family for socialization and common activities.

Other Work areas. The basement is large and contains boxes, cans, and jars; an old TV; and other broken-down electrical equipment besides Robert's workbench, tools, and models described previously. The house has no garage.

Assessment of the Immediate Neighborhood

Neighborhood.   The Fox home is on the outer edge of the neighborhood, built along a main traffic artery leading to the next town. The neighborhood of small homes of about 30 years of age covers some three square miles and the slope of the hill, which starts in the center of town and reaches the top in the area of the Fox home and the doctor's office next door. The neighborhood is orderly and clean. The ages of the inhabitants are mixed. Some of the original owners, like the Foxes, still live there; other houses are occupied by families with children. The number of children per family is rather small, however, owing to the small size of the homes.

Church.   Mrs. Fox's Lutheran church is some six blocks from her home. The distance is too great, and she needs transportation provided by her daughter or a friend.

Transportation, Shopping, Recreational, Medical Facilities.   See community assessment.

Assessment of Interaction Patterns

Common Interests.   Robert and Mrs. Fox live separate lives. Meals and occasional TV watching are the only times they spend together. Mrs. Fox and her daughter both are concerned about Robert's health, and their common interest is to keep up the household as long as possible.

Division of Labor.   The women of the family do the work. The men have a rather parasitic existence. Robert has no responsibilities, and his brother does not offer anything in return for the services he enjoys. He keeps his own money; in fact, he does not have enough, and borrows from his sister and mother after spending too much in the bar. Both women support his alcohol habit and complain bitterly. The daughter, who works full time in an office in town, spends one to two hours with the family and more on weekends. She does most of the cleaning.

Roles.   Mrs. Fox and Robert both are providers, both receiving social security. The money is sufficient, since the home is paid off.

Mrs. Fox takes care of everyone's emotional well-being. Robert takes on the role of the dependent, the spoiled child, and so does his brother.

Mrs. Fox's daughter has taken over the mother role, doing the work that needs to be done in order to make the household function, and she also provides transportation. Only through her can Mrs. Fox interact with the community. She also perpetuates cultural patterns and religious patterns. She takes Mrs. Fox to church, decorates the home for Christmas, bakes cookies for them, and so on.

Assessment of Communication Patterns

Communication.   Mrs. Fox and Robert: Poor. Robert does not initiate conversation. He mumbles and complains. Mrs. Fox uses the few minutes per day she is with him to remind him of what he should be doing. Robert spends most of his time at home secluded in the basement. Robert's health is the main and almost exclusive conversational topic of the two.

Robert and his sister fall into a similar pattern. Robert avoids her also, and she reminds him as much as his mother does of his diet, hygiene, and so on. But since she is gone during the day and removed from the scene, she does address Robert, asking what happened when she was gone. She is trying to show interest in his doings, and at times he responds by showing her the progress he has made with his models.

Mrs. Fox and older son: Communication is nonproductive. Mrs. Fox has ceased to remind him of what he should be doing, since his reaction to this is extreme anger. Mrs. Fox, as a result, complies with his wishes and says few words. At times she inquires how he is doing but does not get much of a response. When in the home, the son keeps to himself or interacts with Robert.

Robert and brother: They have some interests in common—the bar, friends, mechanical inclination, TV shows, and anger at their mother. Robert has deep admiration for his brother. His brother does not put any restrictions on Robert; he does not care about his medical condition but takes him to the bar. They share happenings and express feelings, such as anger. Robert's brother gains self-esteem because Robert follows him.

Emotional Disclosure.   Disclosure of problems happens between the two males and between the two females but not between the two sexes. The mother-daughter relationship used to be more supportive in the past. Now the daughter feels the pressure of responsibilities and complains a lot; the mother feels guilty and depressed and stays quiet rather than burden the daughter with more of her problems. The daughter is quite open with her and expresses her worries openly.

Robert discloses his problems to his brother, whereas his brother communicates only selected bits and pieces of his inner self. He does not bring into the family problems encountered at work or in his own family. The mother often serves as a scapegoat for the anger of both.

Affection.   Affection between the mother and the male family members is not shown. It is covered up by angry feelings. The mother shows affection by doing things for them. She expresses her worries to others. She protects them in spite of their maladaptive coping. The daughter feels anger toward her older brother for being a nuisance and misleading Robert, and for taking advantage of them. She likes Robert and feels hurt about his not wanting to accept her. She blames her brother for that. The mother and daughter feel affection; however, the daughter's feelings are ambivalent. She is angry at her mother for letting herself go and making her work so much. She is fighting these feelings, since she knows at her mother's age this has to be expected.

Fighting and Arguments.   Robert is the most belligerent family member. Arguments between mother and his brother have stopped, since mother keeps quiet. At times tension can be felt, however, and an explosion in the near future is a possibility. Arguments are settled by withdrawal and keeping quiet.

Closeness and Support.   Closeness is present even if not apparent. In emergency situations the members become supportive. This was seen when Robert needed to be hospitalized.

Assessment of Socioeconomic Factors: Income

Income is from social security for both Mrs. Fox and Robert. Mrs. Fox's daughter provides food, household equipment, and other things. There are no monetary worries in the family. Health expenses are covered by Medicaid. Robert gets some pocket money from his check. Mrs. Fox is able to manage the money.

Assessment of Family Health Practices

Medical Services.   The family uses the neighborhood osteopath exclusively. Mrs. Fox has never been hospitalized. Robert has been in a hospital in the next city under care of a specialist five times within the last 10 years. In case of emergencies the neighborhood doctor is consulted, and he will refer the family according to their needs.

Illness Prevention.   Mrs. Fox is strongly aware of the importance of diet, rest, and exercise. As a result of being depressed, she has given up following through with preventive health practices as she did in the past. Trying to remind Robert of their importance has resulted in friction and hurt feelings. Mrs. Fox has retreated to a great extent and only pursues absolutely necessary measures for Robert, such as insulin and diet.

Self-Treatment.   Mrs. Fox visits the doctor only when she cannot handle the illness anymore. She uses herb teas, hot compresses, and special diets to fight ailments. She can use a thermometer and keeps a check on her own and Robert's weight. Hygiene is considered an important aspect of health.

REFERENCES

Archer SE, Fleshman RP: *Community Health Nursing: Patterns and Practice,* ed 2. North Scituate, Duxbury, Mass, 1979.

Duvall EM: *Marriage and Family Development.* Lippincott, Philadelphia, 1977.

Goble F: *The Third Force: The Psychology of Abraham Maslow.* New York, Pocket Books, 1971, pp 37–53.

Mirowski J II, and Ross CE: Minority status, ethnic culture and distress: A comparison of Blacks, Whites, Mexicans and Mexican Americans. *American Journal of Sociology* 86: 479–495, 1980.

Pasquali EA, Alesi IG, Arnold HM, DeBasio N: *Mental Health Nursing: A Bio-Psycho-Cultural Approach.* St Louis, Mosby, 1981.

Smitherman C: *Nursing Actions for Health Promotion.* Philadelphia, FA Davis, 1981.

Tinkham CW, Voorhies EF: *Community Health Nursing: Evolution and Process,* ed 2. New York, Appleton-Century-Crofts, 1977.

World Health Organization. *Constitution: World Health Organization.* Geneva, 1971.

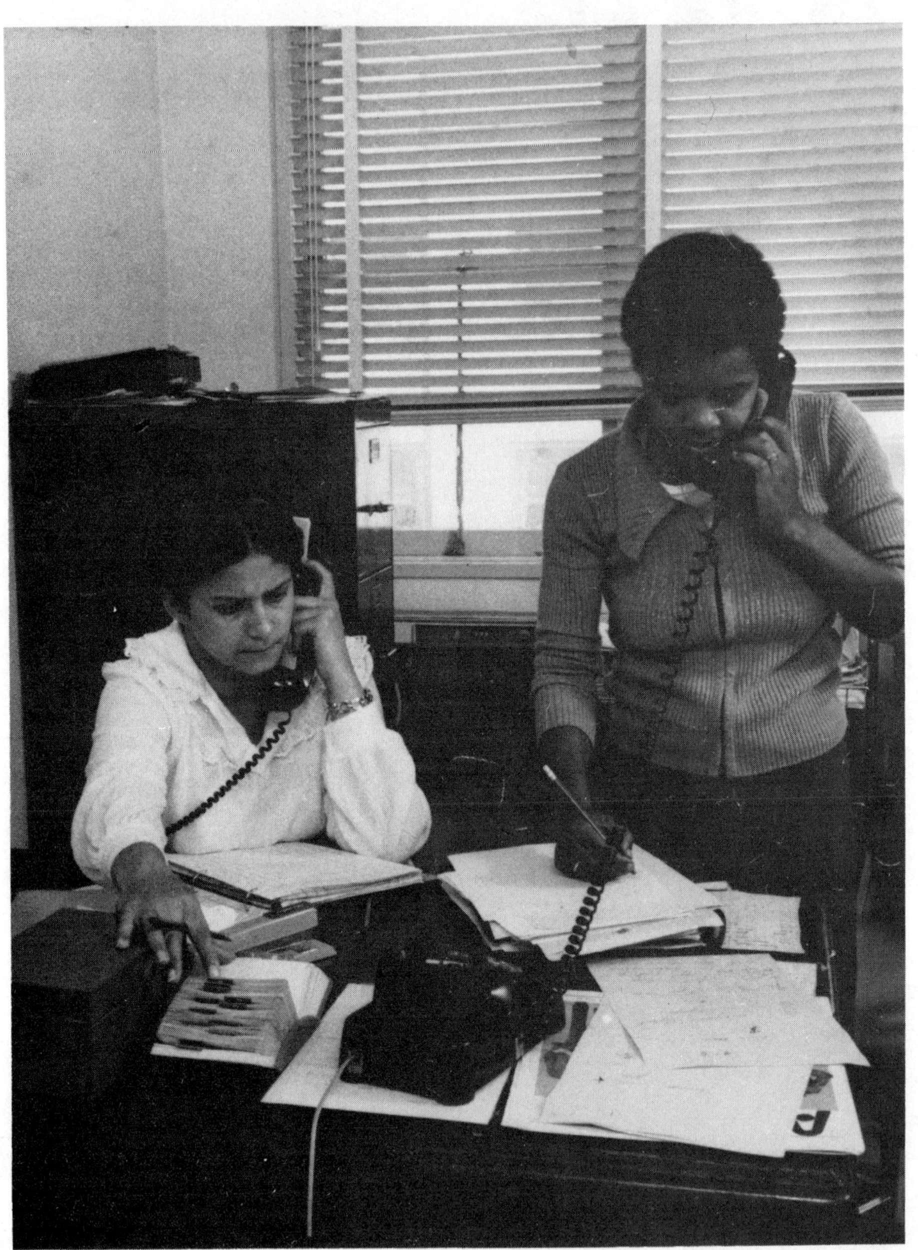

© MICHAL HERON 1981/WOODFIN CAMP & ASSOCIATES

2

Constructing the Care Plan

An assessment consists of a vast amount of material. If it is arranged under the headings proposed in Chapter 1 or filled in on a printed assessment form, it has structure, which helps the nurse to identify the main problem areas while doing the assessment. With experience and skill, it becomes easier to detect relationships between different areas; the assessment reveals a network of factors influencing the client's behavior and attitudes, as well as his or her physical and emotional health.

No area stands by itself. Lack of exercise, for example, may not only mean a weakened physical condition but also may influence the person's emotional well-being. Tension built up that could have been released through exercise, may lead to a need for emotional outlets, so that, for instance, the person may subconsciously set up scenes for marital arguments in an attempt to release that tension. An unmet need for others' respect or affection may play into these dynamics. The guilt produced by yelling at the spouse may throw the person into depression and further reduce his or her willingness to exercise. Thus, as Figure 2-1 indicates, relationships between factors influencing someone's health seem to be cyclical: one area affects the others until the effect again reaches the primary problem area, causing more of a negative effect than it did at first.

It should be understood that the primary problem area is only primary in terms of the *time of diagnosis*. In the above case, for instance, the unmet need of others' esteem might be the initial problem, the root of which may date back years and may in turn stem from a more basic problem, the way in which the client was raised as a child. However, it is not so important for the nurse to assess the root of the problem in the

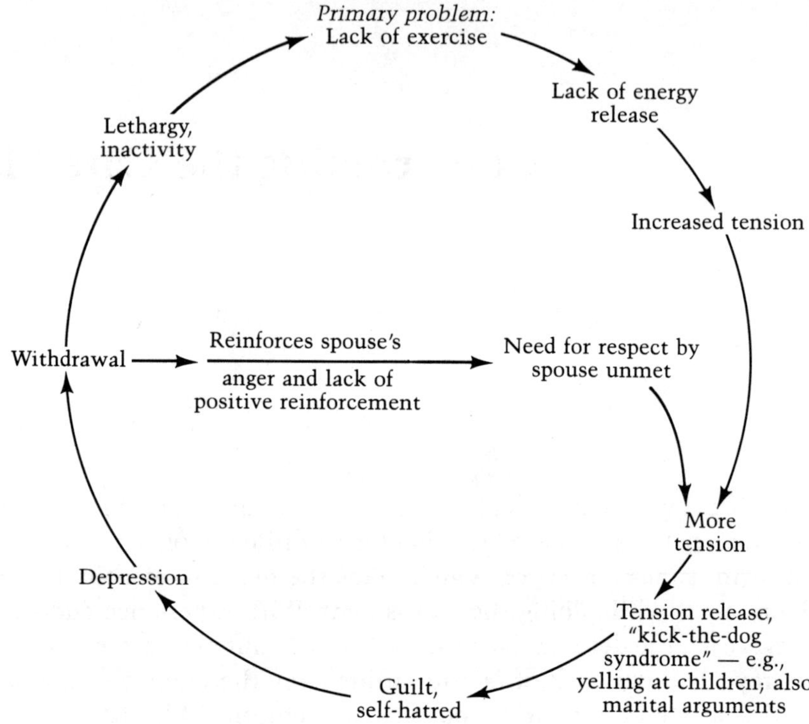

FIGURE 2-1   The cyclical nature of the factors influencing a person's health.

history of the client's life as it is to comprehend its effect on other health areas. If the cyclical nature of such problems is established, a way has to be found by which the cycle can be broken and its devastating effect over time can be halted. In the above example, even if the initial problem, the lack of exercise, is removed, the underlying problem areas will not be corrected, since the damage has left traces in many areas which are no longer related to exercise. Arguments and hurt feelings may have undermined the marital relationship, and the children may exhibit emotional problems such as aggression or inability to concentrate in school. Thus, problems that initially were small reinforce themselves, owing to their cyclical nature, and involve other health areas.

At times community health nurses feel overwhelmed by the scope of problems, reacting to the complexity of these difficulties just as the family in crisis does. The only way to overcome this feeling of helplessness and hopelessness is to organize the assessment data into orderly processes that can be understood. The nurses must use their theoretical knowledge base to ascertain patterns of behavior and relationships between assessment areas. This task is the most difficult one in the nursing process, since information about the family, individuals, and the community must be integrated in order to produce a realistic, workable picture of the family situation. If nurses work in teams, data integration should be done in groups so that different skills and expertise can be applied to the process and the beginning nurse can experience learning instead of frustration.

The end product of such integration of data is a care plan based on a detailed list of the family's problems and strengths. Table 2-1 outlines step by step how the collected assessment data can be ordered and organized into a comprehensive care plan. Let us review each step.

STEP 1: EXAMINING EACH ASSESSMENT SEPARATELY

Step 1 calls for examination of each assessment area separately. Because problems that may be encountered are of different natures and may require

TABLE 2-1 COLLECTING AND ORGANIZING ASSESSMENT DATA INTO A CARE PLAN

Integrating the Data

Step 1: Examine each assessment area separately. Assess fixed problems, avoidable problems, potential problems and strengths.

Step 2: Build a network, connecting the problems of different areas, and assess relationships between them.

Step 3: Recognize orderly patterns.

Step 4: Establish priorities for problems according to their cumulative effect on the health status.

Constructing the Care Plan

Step 5: Word nursing diagnoses.

Step 6: Formulate objectives with a time frame. Assess how strengths can be used to solve problems.

Step 7: Write out a plan for intervention and a teaching plan.

Steps 3, 4, and 7 are planned jointly with the family.

different types of interventions, it is important to categorize these problems:

1.   *Fixed problems* cannot be solved. Nursing care has the aim of adapting to fixed problems by accepting them and by avoiding secondary problems. Fixed problems should be listed together with the other problems they lead to.

2.   *Avoidable problems* are not always totally avoidable, but in most instances they can be modified and rendered less harmful. They are amenable to direct intervention.

3.   *Potential problems* are looked at in terms of future planning. Adaptation is not simply being resigned to the status quo but views the processes as continuing. The client needs to learn to expect what will happen and to adjust to changes by anticipating them and preparing for them.

An example of Step 1 for Robert Fox and his family is shown in Table 2-2, using assessment data from Chapter 1. Because readers are not able to observe in person, our example is very detailed but necessary for complete understanding. In reality, a nurse may need to write down a lesser amount of detail in order to arrive at the same result.

STEP 2: DIAGRAMMING THE NETWORK

In this step, after all problems and strengths are listed and their nature determined, the problems are integrated into a comprehensive framework with the help of a diagram. This step is the most difficult, since it demands systematic thinking about the relationships between the problems and the different areas. The nurse needs to know theory in order to comprehend the why of symptoms and behaviors, and also needs a certain amount of creativity and a clear understanding of reality. These qualities are essential for the construction of a conceptual framework that is the basis for broad understanding and comprehensive intervention. The closer the framework is to reality, the more likely it is that intervention will work. The better the nurse's theoretical understanding, the more likely it is that the conceptual framework will be workable. One of the major problems in nursing is the "hit or miss" nature of interventions; too often, an intervention is simply a good guess.

TABLE 2-2 LIST OF PROBLEMS AND STRENGTHS FOR ROBERT FOX AND FAMILY: PRIMARY PREVENTION

Key: FP = Fixed problem
AP = Avoidable problem
PP = Potential problem
S = Strength

ASSESSMENT DATA	FP	AP	PP	S	EXPLANATION
Robert—History: Physical					
Prematurity			x		Possible overprotection
Mild mental retardation—lack of special training	x	x			Influences diverse areas of daily living: • gainful employment • independence status • decision making
Anger outbreaks		x			Negative effect on family relationship, ability to be gainfully employed
Basic math and reading skills				x	Increased chance for occupation
Diabetes	x	x			Fixed problem since there is no cure. Physical and emotional effects can be modified or eliminated.
Obesity		x			Dangerous physical effect also emotional effect.
Neuropathy	x		x		Pain and weakness not avoidable. Progressive nature threat to security—gait stability.
Suspicious, noncommunicative manner		x		x	Problem influences teaching effectiveness. Protects Robert's ego by withdrawing from potentially harmful people.
Mrs. Fox—History: Physical					
Age 92, failing health			x		Diminishing physical functions possible threat to safety.
Widow of many years				x	Ability to cope in hard times. Independence.

TABLE 2-2 *(continued)*

ASSESSMENT DATA	FP	AP	PP	S	EXPLANATION
Forgetfulness	x		x		Negative influence on Robert's diabetic regime. Potential problem of safety.
Hypertension	?	x			May be avoidable if positively modified by medication and stress avoidance.
Refusal to take medications		x		x	Prevents hypertension management. Shows determination, belief in own resources.
Thin, fragile appearance			x		Decreased resistance to disease.
Dental prostheses			x		Difficulties chewing—nutritional status.
Alertness, coordination, productive thinking				x	No functional impairment.
Weakness in left arm	x	?			Impairment of arm function; effect on emotional status, possibly safety. Possibly may improve with exercise.
Depressed mood		x			May be self-perpetuating.
Robert—Diet and Fluids					
Unclear understanding of diet in relation to diabetes		x			Does not take any responsibility for eating habits.
Not concerned with meal preparation or kinds of food he eats	?	?			Unclear whether intelligence and motivation present to get interested in taking some responsibility for food preparation.
Diet transgressions—snacks, drinks, alcoholic beverages		x			Problem serves other needs. Robert is resistant to change lifestyle and give up psychological rewards.
Foods brought in from several sources—daughter, neighbors, friends.		x			Main suppliers of food need to be informed.
Insufficient awareness of these people with regard to Robert's diabetes				x	Friends and neighbors show concern.

ASSESSMENT DATA	FP	AP	PP	S	EXPLANATION
Home food preparation less conscientious due to Mother's failing health, depression, and forgetfulness		x			Control of diabetes more difficult.
Meaning of food to Robert	x				Habits hard to change unless Robert's friends help. Food has social meaning to Robert. Not likely to give it up.
Liking for sweets		x			Harmful. Will go to the people who give him sweets or buy them.
Fast eating		x			Wants to avoid mother.
Need for teaching of diabetic diet and 4 food groups		x			Has to show motivation— need for solving emotional problems prior to teaching.
Mrs. Fox—Diet and Fluids					
Unfamiliar with four food groups			x		May influence variety of diet and adherence to diabetic diet difficult.
Is knowledgeable about diet balancing				x	Awareness can be used in teaching plan
Keeps sugar out of the home				x	
Concerned about Robert's health status				x	May be willing to make changes
Eats very little. Has no appetite		x			Nutritional needs smaller when old. Lack of appetite probably based on physical and emotional exhaustion, hopelessness.
Vitamin supplement				x	Listens to doctor's advice.
Difficulties chewing			x		May further reduce appetite due to limited variety of foods.
No snacks			x		May be getting less than nutritional needs.

TABLE 2-2 (continued)

ASSESSMENT DATA	FP	AP	PP	S	EXPLANATION
Three meals, eating in kitchen				x	Is programmed to eat at certain times of the day.
Loss of taste for vegetables. Possible loss of taste due to old age	x		x		May lead to vitamin deficiency. Loss of taste may further reduce appetite.
Still has some foods she likes to eat: bread, milk products				x	Can be used in modifying diet to make it more attractive.
Food has lost meaning		x			Due to unpleasantness of communication with Robert during meals. Related to depression.
Robert—Activity and Rest Pattern					
Gainfully employed in the past in friend's trucking company				x	Potential for employment. Able to take on some responsibility; dependability is uncertain.
Decreasing physical strength	x				Influences emotional well-being.
Exercise—daily walks to town				x	
Decrease in exercise compared to time of employment		x			Weight gain. Decreased physical and emotional well-being.
Need for teaching in area		x			Motivation gained possibly by dealing with emotional needs.
Sufficient rest, no problem with sleep				x	
Sleeping routine may interfere with diabetic regime: hard to arouse in morning; goes back to bed after insulin and breakfast.			x		Stress on Mrs. Fox. Inactivity may increase need for insulin. Also lends to weight gain.
Skills, hobbies, intelligence level impressive in certain areas				x	Source of self-esteem. Potential for training for other type of employment.

TABLE 2-2 (continued)

ASSESSMENT DATA	FP	AP	PP	S	EXPLANATION
Mrs. Fox—Activity and Rest Pattern					
Decreasing level of involvement in houshold and garden; increasing dependency	x	x			Possibly partially due to emotional factors. This could be modified—age component needs to be adapted to.
Change in sleep pattern		x			Probably due to inactivity, depression, difficulties adapting to physical limitations.
Lack of exercise: has given up gardening, walks, household work		x			Seems capable of doing more. Emotional factors involved.
Robert—Life Enjoyment and Satisfaction					
No problems with physical needs				x	
Withdrawal of interest in women			x		Possibly resulting from and adding to low self-esteem.
No safety problems				x	
Refusal to go to church, possible rejection of religion			x		Creates value friction between Robert and Mrs. Fox. Significant help in coping not available.
Financial security: social security and family support				x	No problems.
Sources of self-esteem • hobbies				x	
• social interaction		x		x	Emotional benefits but danger to physical health due to friends offering food and drinks.
Coping with social stigma by withdrawal			x	x	Effective self-protection, barrier to trusting helping people.
Depression evidenced by anger outbreaks, withdrawal—increased since physical condition has deteriorated		x			Mostly evident at home.

TABLE 2-2 (continued)

ASSESSMENT DATA	FP	AP	PP	S	EXPLANATION
Rebellion against dependency		x		x	Leads to noncompliance. Wants to gain independence—motivated to change.
Frustration and disappointment with goals for future • drums • loss of job		x			Depression. Inability to see remaining strengths.
Does not feel accepted by family		x			Rebellious, angry. Needs recognition and positive reinforcement.
Mrs. Fox—Life Enjoyment and Satisfaction					
Able to handle household partially; good coordination				x x	
Failing eyesight and memory; need for teaching safety precautions			x		Increases dependency. Security threatened.
Self-esteem derived through autonomy and independence		x			Physical deterioration leads to depression. Keeps sons in dependent state.
Purpose for living: to take care of Robert		x			Inability to reach goal leads to depression and worry.
Inability to adapt to natural physical changes due to age		x			No planning for future has been done.
Religious belief				x	Goes to church regularly.
Robert and Mrs. Fox— Social Support System					
Mutual support within family				x	
Daughter is willing to support family				x	
Robert does not take any part in supporting mother; affection not usually apparent		x			Affects Mrs. Fox's emotional status.

TABLE 2-2 (continued)

ASSESSMENT DATA	FP	AP	PP	S	EXPLANATION
Trusting relationship between brother and Robert		x		x	Helps Robert emotionally. Brother shows no concern for Robert's physical problems.
Mrs. Fox used to be center of family support, now daughter is taking over. Daughter feels overburdened		x		x	Seems to foster dependence in the sons—creates resistance.
Many friends and concerned people in town				x	
Robert has created own friendship circle				x	
Doctor is part of the friendship circle				x	Has been very helpful to family; his advice is usually followed.
Robert—Stress					
Stress due to frustration • deterioration of health • growing dependence		x			Result of authority conflict and noncompliance—perpetuate problem by increasing dependence.
Nonproductive coping		x			Anger, association with friends in town—eating and drinking.
Mrs. Fox—Stress					
Deteriorating physical health	x	x			Process cannot be halted, but Mrs. Fox needs to learn to adapt.
Fear of losing control over self and Robert or Robert's brother		x			Communication breakdown and hurt feelings.
Need for stress teaching		x			Recognition of own symptoms and needs understanding of Robert's behavior through teaching.

TABLE 2-2 (continued)

ASSESSMENT DATA	FP	AP	PP	S	EXPLANATION
Robert—Preventive Medical, Dental, and Eye Care					
Medical care good				x	
Doctor using community resource for problems beyond his control				x	
Needs dental appointment			x		Possible tooth decay.
Needs eye appointment		x			Insufficient eyesight, difficulties with hobbies
Anger at medical doctor			x		Resistance to advice.
Satisfactory hygiene; resistance when reminded by Mrs. Fox			x	x	Robert is increasingly hard to handle. Without a reminder, would not shower.
Mrs. Fox—Preventive Medical, Dental, and Eye Care					
Regular eye care				x	
Regular medical care				x	
Dental: May need plates adjusted; problems chewing			x		Possibly related to lack of appetite.
Hygiene excellent				x	
Refrigeration of foods not enforced sufficiently			x		Danger of food poisoning.

**TABLE 2-3. LIST OF ASSESSMENT FOR
SECONDARY AND TERTIARY PREVENTION**

ASSESSMENT DATA	FP	AP	PP	S	EXPLANATION
Robert					
Uncontrolled diabetes		x			Needs better understanding of disease—motivate prior to teaching.
Neuropathy	x				
Possible retinopathy			x		
Pain in legs	x	x			Adaptation can be achieved. Weight loss probably beneficial.
Interference with function	x				Inability to perform previous job.
Emotional reaction		x			
Treatment and equipment: Mrs. Fox and daughter are informed				x	
Difficulties administering treatment efficiently		x			Time pressure and Mrs. Fox's physical limitations.
Robert's potential unused		x			
No responsibility given		x			
Mrs. Fox					
Old age	x				
Hypertension; arteriosclerosis		x			Needs teaching; prevent deterioration.
Recent noncompliance with medical regime; medication refused		x			Has not seen doctor.
Emotional reaction—depression		x			
Interference with function	x	x			Modification possible. Adaptation to limitation.
Physical condition uncontrolled		x			

TABLE 2-4. LIST OF THE FAMILY: ASSESSMENT OF OTHER INFLUENTIAL FAMILY MEMBERS

ASSESSMENT DATA	FP	AP	PP	S	EXPLANATION
Mrs. Fox's daughter					
Great support and in household				x	
Daily visits				x	Increased security.
Mrs. Fox's older son					
Dependent, alcoholic		x			Leads parasitic existence.
Resists mother's authority		x			Influences Robert's noncompliance negatively.
Does not take responsibility; Mrs. Fox supports dependence, takes care of his physical needs—indirectly supports drinking habit		x x			
Visits frequently—when he wants to be taken care of		x			Mrs. Fox resents, but does not discourage.
Gets money support from sister and mother		x			Increases dependency.
Home					
Satisfactory condition and cleanliness				x	
Yard reflects Mrs. Fox's problem with ill health			x		May affect her emotional well-being.
Living area sufficient in size				x	
Family closeness expressed by many photographs				x	
Bedrooms—satisfactory; cluttered, but reasonably clean				x	
Allow for individuality				x	Mother does not interfere with Robert's collection of models and magazines.
Bathroom and kitchen functional				x	
Kitchen cluttered and somewhat untidy			x		Influences safety.
Basement functional and safe				x	Serves Robert's needs.

TABLE 2-4 (continued)

ASSESSMENT DATA	FP	AP	PP	S	EXPLANATION
Interaction Patterns					
Little communication between Mrs. Fox and Robert		x			Affects Mrs. Fox's emotional well-being. Robert looks for gratifications elsewhere.
Mrs. Fox and daughter domineering		x			Reduce Robert's autonomy—resentment.
Foster Robert's and brother's dependency		x			Both men take advantage of it but resent it by being angry and uncooperative.
Mrs. Fox and daughter communicate well				x	
Daughter complains a lot—much pressure owing to responsibility. Resents uninvolvement of men. Tension, quarrels		x			Mrs. Fox made to feel that she is a burden. Fear that daughter may leave her.
The men cope by withdrawing and supporting one another		x			Further deterioration of communication.
Division of Labor					
Unequal distribution; women carry all responsibility		x			Resentment and anger.
Mother–daughter role reversal			x		Daughter feels overburdened.
Increasing dependency on daughter of whole family	x	x			Mother's dependency natural. Daughter reinforces mother's handling of the men—perpetuates situation.
Daughter took over authoritarian position			x	x	Needed to run family. Creates resentment in the men.
Daughter now responsible for cultural and religious pattern			x		Adds to burden.

ASSESSMENT DATA	FP	AP	PP	S	EXPLANATION
Communication Patterns					
Robert–Mrs. Fox: Robert avoids Mrs. Fox, withdraws, gets angry, complains, mumbles, or insults. Mrs. Fox keeps reminding him of duties and diabetes regime; threatens		x			Needs of both do not get met. Disapprove of one another; resentment.
Robert–sister: Same pattern as above. Sister meets some of Robert's needs, shows interest for his hobby. Communication deteriorating as sister takes on mother's role more and more		x		x	Initially warm feelings between the two. Positive aspects still kept up. Response to pressure to comply is same as when mother does it.
Mrs. Fox–older son: Nonproductive. Son shows extreme anger and resentment. Mother withdraws		x			Consequences of dependency relationship of son. Affects Mrs. Fox's emotional well-being.
Daughter–older son: Same as above.		x			
Robert–older son: Friendship, warmth, teasing friendliness. Robert admires him			x	x	Family member Robert listens to. Potentially bad influence if older son's interactions are not in line with medical regime of Robert. Relationship is source of self-esteem for both.
Emotional Disclosure					
Mother–daughter used to be extensive. Now mother is holding back—daughter complains and makes mother feel like a burden. Mother does not want to burden her with more problems		x	x		Both do not meet their needs—communication breakdown.

TABLE 2-4 (continued)

ASSESSMENT DATA	FP	AP	PP	S	EXPLANATION
Robert discloses to brother; brother discloses partially. Does not share own marital problems				x	Beneficial for both.
Mother serves as scapegoat		x			Unified power against mother—less compliance.
Affection					
Mrs. Fox does things for family. Expresses worries to friends				x	
Protects them—protects maladaptive coping		x			
Much resentment: daughter–older son; sons–mother and daughter		x			
Mutual caring present in emergency situations—getting Robert to the hospital				x	
Fighting and Arguments					
Robert belligerent. Keeps quiet as long as mother keeps quiet		x			Emotional tension unreleased.
Settle arguments by withdrawing		x		x	Decreased chance of physical harm.
Socioeconomic Factors					
No problem				x	
Family Health Practices					
Awareness of importance of diet, rest, exercise				x	Only accepted by women.
Self-treatment as much as possible before seeing doctor			x	x	May wait too long. No unnecessary doctor's visits.

TABLE 2-5. LIST OF PROBLEMS AND STRENGTHS FOR ROBERT FOX AND FAMILY: RELATED COMMUNITY FACTORS

ASSESSMENT DATA	FP	AP	PP	S	EXPLANATION
Small town. People know each other, are concerned				x	
Work opportunities for Robert limited			x		Needs transportation to next town.
Recreational facilities adequate				x	
Conservative attitude			x		Possible resistance to change—employment of Robert.
Lack of cultural attraction. Bar is substitute		x			Influences lifestyle, especially for men in the village. Robert is tempted.
Active practice of religion—many churches				x	Generally attitude of concern for each other.
No hospitals in town			x		Transportation needed.
Activity group for the mentally ill—social stigma—conservative attitude of people prevents Robert from joining			x		
Closeness of downtown area			x	x	Stimulation and temptation for Robert.
Education level of the population rather low			x		May be unaware of Robert's physical problems.
Older population predominant in downtown area				x	Have seen Robert grow up. Accept him.
Immediate Neighborhood					
No threat to safety				x	
Friendly neighbors				x	
Need for transportation for church, shopping, hospital, and so on	x				Increase of dependency on daughter.
Doctor's office next door				x	

There are two misconceptions about client care that are widely applied. The first is the belief that if an intervention has worked for one client it will also work for another; many times this does not hold true. The second is that teaching is the panacea for all problems and that "if only people knew facts they would do better." Thus, nurses often categorize problems and corresponding solutions in their minds, and care plans consist of nothing more than matching the two. Since they believe the only reason a client is not practicing optimal health care is lack of knowledge, their solution is simply to teach, covering all areas in which the client has problems. Such a procedure is simple and is practiced internationally, and the nursing profession has been very efficient in refusing to realize that it does not work. Diabetics still do not follow their diets, obese people do not lose weight, heart patients forget to do their exercises; and many nurses themselves smoke, consume too much alcohol, and do not get enough rest. Should they not know best?

Constructing such a conceptual framework is time consuming and demands skills not previously taught in many schools, but if done carefully it may work. Initially, the procedure takes time and effort. In the long run, however, it saves time, error, frustration, and, above all, money.

The network of problems shown in Figures 2-2 and 2-3 is a result of system thinking. Traditional thinking in terms of linear relationships simply does not lead to results in community nursing. Even for hospital care, it is evident that clients with the same diagnosis react differently to the same treatment. In community nursing, intervening variables are of still greater importance, for the nurse must deal not only with strict medical problems but with the complex problem of optimal health, which involves physical and emotional factors. Just as cancer does not seem to be caused by a single agent, optimal health too is determined by many factors. It is the interaction of these factors and their effect upon each other that the nurse needs to understand. A diagram (such as the example of Figures 2-2 and 2-3) should be constructed as a visual aid to understanding. Nurses need to be able to think such a diagram through and follow the lines of relationships; yet they must realize none of the lines can be designated as strictly right or wrong, that the same problem can be attacked from different angles and many interventions may lead to similar results. Experience will show which ways are the most effective, as nurses come to recognize similarities of patterns between cases.

The drawing of the conceptual framework that the nurse devises must be shared with clients, who often will be able to point out relationships

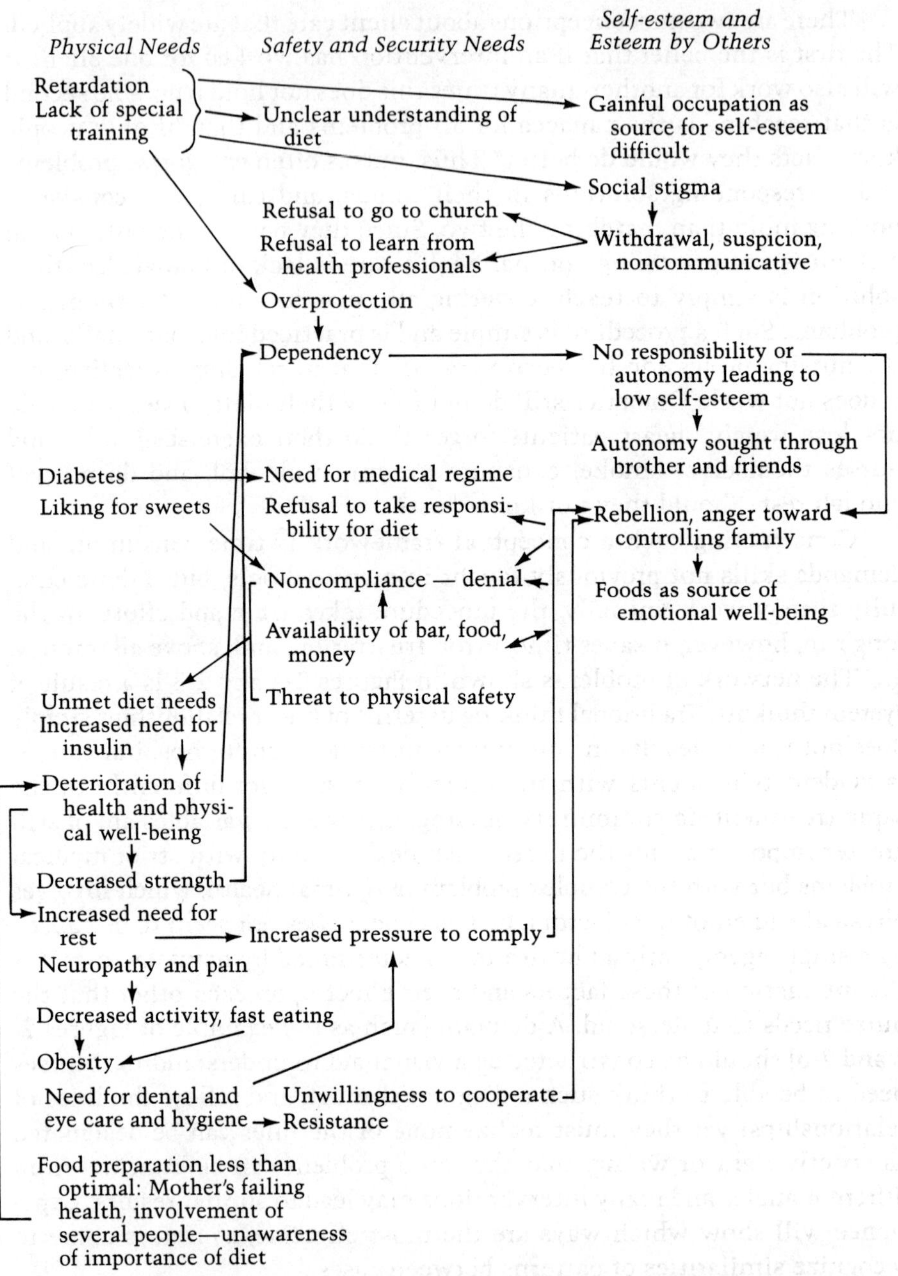

FIGURE 2-2.   Network of problems organized according to need categories—Robert Fox.

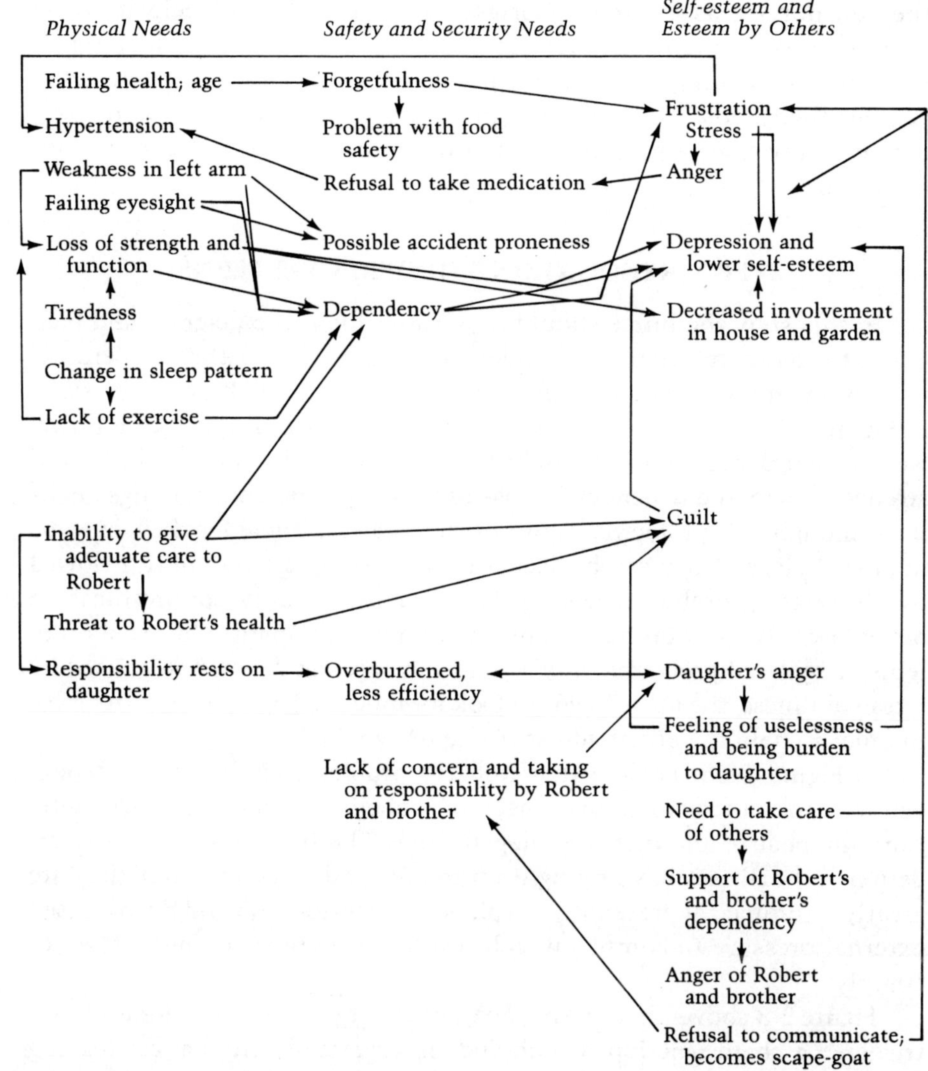

FIGURE 2-3.   Network of problems organized according to need categories—Mrs. Fox.

they do not see as accurate. Correcting these early will help to avoid unnecessary interventions later. In addition, the family may be of great value in establishing priorities for problems, since they know best what worries them most. Even if their opinions are different from the nurse's, whatever the family perceives as the main problem should get primary attention.

STEP 3: RECOGNIZING ORDERLY PATTERNS

In this step, the nurse should look carefully at the diagram and pick out patterns in an attempt to understand the nature of the problems. If most problems are related to one particular problem (such as "depression" in Figure 2-3), this is likely to be the key one. In the example that follows, we see that depression is brought on by deterioration of health, loss of strength, increased dependency, loss of function, and guilt feelings about it. Although the problems may not be totally avoidable, they may be improved; dependency can be decreased and deterioration of health slowed by eliminating problems leading to it, such as family communication breakdown. If a key problem is brought on predominantly by fixed problems or by fixed problems only, such as in cases of depression caused by terminal illness, the nurse needs to look for modifiers, the client's strengths, in order to help the client adjust to the unavoidable.

In Figure 2-2 it is clear that Robert's problems circle around dependency—lack of responsibility, anger and rebellion, noncompliance, deteriorating health, and increased dependency. The fixed problems of retardation and diabetes have brought on the dependency cycle, but they are greatly reinforced at present by his physical deterioration and by increased external pressure to comply, which results in more anger and refusal to comply.

Figure 2-3 shows that in Mrs. Fox's case her physical deterioration has triggered a chain reaction, which ends in practically all changes leading to stress and depression; it can be easily understood why depression in turn would help to further weaken her physical condition. These dynamics make it questionable whether Mrs. Fox's physical deterioration is actually a fixed problem. If it were triggered by a multifactoral process, it might well be possible to halt the process and prevent it from further reducing her strength.

The bottom half of Figure 2-3 shows how reactions and behaviors of other family members influence Mrs. Fox's depression. Putting Mrs. Fox in the position of scapegoat makes her feel guilty. It supposedly is her fault that the daughter works so hard, that Robert's diabetes is out of control. It is her fault, they say, that Robert's brother has remained in the role of a child and has no autonomy, that he is drinking and is losing his wife. He has the right to take it out on her and demand that she take care of him. If Mrs. Fox fails, he is angry.

Where can these cycles be broken? If, for example, Robert's friendship circle and the bar were removed and Robert had no chance for diet transgression, his diabetes problem might improve. However, such a solution is not realistic.

A traditional nurse, following doctor's orders, would have visited the house, bringing some booklets and diet information, and would have taught Robert and Mrs. Fox the importance of a diabetic diet. Mrs. Fox would have listened politely, answered the nurse's questions, and at the end of the hour been able to write down a menu for Robert, under the supervision of the nurse. Meanwhile Robert would have sat on the couch, brooding and mumbling from time to time. The nurse would have stressed to him innumerable times how harmful sweets were and how continuing to visit the bar would put him in the hospital again. Robert would have nodded and sighed, which would start Mrs. Fox thinking about doing some special cooking during the next few days until the impact of the nurse's visit had worn off—and so Robert would have merrily continued his daily routine.

Figures 2-2 and 2-3 show why such a traditional intervention is not effective. Many more factors are involved. Robert does not transgress because of lack of knowledge, but because he *needs* to for his emotional well-being. Unless he feels like a worthy human being, life is not worth living. In the past, his lifestyle has rewarded him socially and emotionally, but changes have occurred and he now suffers physical backlashes. He seems unwilling to give up his emotional rewards for better physical health. He clings with desperation to the old routine and struggles bitterly against change. Mrs. Fox, too, feels herself overcome by changes she cannot handle. Indeed she feels doubly burdened because she not only feels the impact of her own weakening physical condition but also the changes affecting Robert. It seems that her caring for Robert has kept her strong and well for so many years. Now she is losing control over herself and over Robert. She senses that her life will come to an end before long, and she sees that without her strong leadership the family functions poorly. She cannot relax and retire but instead is driven by anxiety. In a desperate attempt to change the son's lifestyle she keeps reminding him of how he should be taking care of himself, not realizing that her nagging has the opposite effect.

STEP 4: ESTABLISHING PRIORITIES FOR PROBLEMS

In this step, a list of priorities is set up. The family should help the nurse determine the accuracy of the findings and set priorities for the problems. The key problems will be those that are caused by most other problems—and in the drawing have most arrows leading to them—but the problems that need to be considered first priority are those that cause most other problems and have most arrows leading *away* from them. If a problem that leads to several other problems is treated first in a care plan, the results of care are likely to show up sooner. If high-priority problems are fixed problems, however, clients first need to learn to cope with them and use their inner strengths before turning attention to secondary problems.

Figures 2-2 and 2-3 indicate which problems seem most important—namely, those that cause most other problems:

For Robert:
  Fixed problems—retardation, diabetes
  Avoidable problems—dependency, rebellion and anger, noncompliance, deterioration of health

For Mrs. Fox:
  Fixed problems—old age, loss of strength, failing eyesight
  Avoidable problems—dependency (can be modified), frustration, depression, guilt, anxiety, feeling of uselessness

Among these problems the community nurse needs to determine which are primary and which mere consequences of these primary problems. In Robert's case, the primary problems are retardation and diabetes. However, previously Robert's adaptation to these problems was satisfactory and his life was in a reasonable balance of health and happiness. The problem that disturbed this equilibrium was the deterioration of his health, and it is likely that Mrs. Fox's loss of function and strength was the determining factor. It is therefore reasonable to consider Mrs. Fox's deterioration of health the primary problem. However, Mrs. Fox's getting old is a fixed problem; rather than attempt to solve this unsolvable problem, a care plan should include measures to help her adapt to it. Since Mrs. Fox's depression is brought on by most other problems (deterioration of her health; her interaction with Robert, which stimulates his noncompliance; her inability to keep control over Robert's diabetic regime), it should be considered a key problem. Robert's key problem lies within the noncompliance–dependency–anger cycle, which is accelerated by deteriorating health, his primary problem. All other problems in Figure 2-2 are closely associated with the cycle.

The problem list is as follows:

Mrs. Fox:
1. Primary problems: old age, loss of strength, and failing eyesight.
2. Associated problems: increased dependency, frustration, guilt, anxiety, feeling of uselessness.
3. Key problem: depression (resulting from fixed primary problem and others).

Robert:
1. Primary problem: deterioration of health.
2. Associated problems: diabetes, retardation, obesity, communication breakdown, etc.
3. Key problems: noncompliance, dependency, anger.

New problems resulting from changes are as follows:

Mrs. Fox:
- anger; refusal to take medication
- forgetfulness; questionable food safety
- change in sleep patterns; tiredness
- lack of exercise
- communication breakdown
- increased need for control

Previous problems now accelerated due to changes are as follows:

Robert:
- difficulty finding a gainful occupation
- withdrawal and suspicion
- need to seek autonomy through friends
- need for food as emotional gratification
- insufficient exercise
- inefficient diet preparation
- cutting off communication with family

STEP 5: WORD NURSING DIAGNOSES

After completing the planning procedure this far, nurses are ready to go through the usual steps of setting up a care plan, using as tools the list of family strengths and the problem list. In wording nursing diagnoses, step 5, nurses should not be preoccupied so much with finding the correct "official" expression in order to make it sound professional as they should be with avoiding writing down any problem on a care plan without understanding its exact nature, the factors leading up to it, and the factors resulting from it. Since no problem stands on its own, each diagnosis, too, has a relationship to all the others.

Table 2-6 indicates the word diagnoses according to priority in the Fox example.

STEP 6: FORMULATING OBJECTIVES

In this step, diagnoses, with the help of related problems and family strengths, are integrated and modeled into a set of objectives. The objectives are a reflection of the nurse's ideal picture of what should happen. They need to be realistic with regard to possible interventions and time frame required to meet the objectives. Experience will tell the nurse how much can realistically be achieved within a certain time frame, within a certain number of visits, and with the help of the limited resources of the family and the nurse. Again, working in teams presents a distinct advantage, especially for the beginning community nurse.

Table 2-7 lists family strengths that the nurse should be aware of and utilize in formulating objectives and a care plan.

STEP 7: THE TREATMENT PLAN

Nursing actions follow as a natural consequence of understanding diagnoses and objectives. They should be discussed with the family and agreed upon by them, so that they have a clear picture of a time schedule and realistic expectation about what and when changes will happen. The family should also be told what input and effort is expected of them to make these changes happen.

Table 2-8 is an example of the nursing objectives and treatment plan for the Foxes.

All family members (including daughter and son) should be knowledgeable about and follow satisfactory health habits, as shown in Table 2-9.

The teaching plan for those areas of primary prevention is presented in Chapter 4.

TABLE 2-6 NURSING DIAGNOSES ORDERED ACCORDING TO PRIORITY

1. Mrs. Fox shows symptoms of depression secondary to failing health and eyesight. Depression is evidenced by
   - Expression of feeling of worthlessness
   - Expression of guilt
   - Expression of frustration, anxiety
   - Change in sleep patterns
   - Chronic exhaustion
   - Decreased appetite
   - Lack of energy to perform housework
2. Robert's diabetes is no longer under control; related to noncompliance with medical regime as evidenced by
   - 3+ and 4+ urine
   - Weight gain
   - Neighbors' account of seeing Robert eating and drinking in town
   - Angry resistance to restrictions imposed by Mrs. Fox
3. Inefficient coping of Mrs. Fox with aging process and hypertension. This is evidenced by
   - Unwillingness to follow medical regime
   - Expressed frustration due to loss of function
4. Communication breakdown between all family members, except Robert and his brother, as evidenced by
   - Anger and withdrawal of Robert
   - Continuing pressuring and nagging of Mrs. Fox with regard to Robert's and his brother's lifestyles
   - Refusal of the men to take on responsibilities
   - Mrs. Fox's withdrawal from daughter owing to daughter's complaints about being overburdened
5. Noncompliance of Robert with medical regime secondary to rebellion and denial, as evidenced by his
   - Accepting food and drinks from friends
   - Refusing responsibility for diet regime
   - Unfavorable sleep and rest patterns
   - Refusal to see dentist or eye doctor
6. Dependency and lack of responsibility of Robert secondary to overprotection.
7. Unmet need for self-esteem and esteem by others (Robert) secondary to loss of gainful employment, increased dependency, failing health, as evidenced by his
   - Needing food for emotional gratification
   - Need to seek autonomy away from home
8. Robert's difficulty with forming trusting relationship secondary to negative experiences owing to social stigma of his handicap. This possibly results in block to teaching and denying him access to religious practices.
9. Potential problem of safety secondary to Mrs. Fox's forgetfulness and loss of physical strength.

TABLE 2-7 FAMILY STRENGTHS RELATED TO NURSING DIAGNOSES AS LISTED IN TABLE 2-6

NURSING DIAGNOSES	FAMILY STRENGTHS
1	Satisfactory living conditions Good medical care, eye care Religion Previous independence and belief in own resources Mental alertness, intelligence Remaining function, good coordination Good relationship with doctor Concerned friends and neighbors Support from daughter Routine meal times, preferred foods No financial worries
2	Routine meal times at home No sweets in the house Mrs. Fox's daughter's concern about Robert's health Concerned neighbors Mrs. Fox's basic understanding of diabetes and diet Positive aspects of interpersonal relationship between Robert and sister
3	Previous coping when husband died Independence and self-sufficiency Remaining mental and physical function Religion Social and family support Daughter's help in household No financial worries
4	Robert's dislike of dependency Robert's trust relationship with brother Positive aspects of relationship between Robert and sister Family concern for Robert Robert's abilities and skills
5	Dislike of dependency of Robert Rebellion Robert's social skills Positive aspects of relationship between Robert and sister Permission for individuality
6	Withdrawal from harmful interaction with people Friendship circle Social skills Hobbies and skills Satisfactory living conditions Trust relationship with brother

TABLE 2-7 *(continued)*

NURSING DIAGNOSES	FAMILY STRENGTHS
7	Concern of family and neighbors and friends for Robert's well-being Good relationship with medical doctor in the past Regular medical check-ups for Robert Positive aspects of relationship between Robert and sister Robert's dislike of dependency
8	Social skills of Robert Trust relationship with brother and friends Positive response of Robert to recognition of his talents
9	Satisfactory living condition Concerns of family and friends Alertness and coordination

TABLE 2-8 NURSING OBJECTIVES AND TREATMENT PLAN

OBJECTIVES	NURSING ACTIONS
Diagnosis 1: Mrs. Fox's Depression *Objectives:* Short-term (after two visits	
1. Mrs. Fox will openly express her feelings of hopelessness, guilt, and anger related to her own condition and Robert's behavior.	Build a trust relationship, listen, help put problems in proper perspective. Stay away from giving advice. Instead listen to client.
2. Mrs. Fox will express the importance of diet and exercise for physical and emotional well-being.	Explain that depression is a natural reaction to events that are beyond control. Explain the progressive nature of depression and its relationship to physical well-being. Gently suggest diet and exercise as initial intervening measures.
3. Mrs. Fox will outline strengths that have helped her cope with depression in the past.	Reestablish some belief in herself by outlining strengths such as previous independence, remaining abilities, and so on. Let Mrs. Fox think of the ways she had coped when her husband died. What is different now? Which strengths and abilities does she still have?

TABLE 2-8 *(continued)*

OBJECTIVES	NURSING ACTIONS
Objectives: Intermediate (after 10 visits)	
4. Mrs. Fox will have set up a plan of daily activities which takes into account her abilities and uses resources (daughter, Robert, neighbors, and so on) without overtaxing them.	Joint family meetings, all involved helping people included. List all tasks that need to be done daily and from time to time. Set up a schedule (written) when tasks are to be done and by whom. Explore everyone's abilities and willingness to help. Discuss situation with Robert's brother. Discuss limits that should be set. Make hospitality conditional on his input in the labor distribution. Express to Robert that his help is needed and appreciated, exert mild pressure only and give much positive reinforcement. Include in plan who is responsible for transportation to provide preventive eye and dental care for Mrs. Fox, also to make it possible for her to go to church—for example, mobilize church members to take her rather than daughter.
Objectives: Long-term (by termination)	
5. Mrs. Fox will express a positive outlook on the future. She will accept necessary help and will contribute whatever she can to the daily routine.	Keep exploring her feelings and her emotional problems about becoming dependent. Help her find worthwhile activities to substitute for the ones she can no longer do—for example, include her in a church group working for a bazaar.
6. Mrs. Fox will accept increasing dependency as a natural process of aging. She will find comfort in satisfaction about what she has achieved in her life, in the affection of her family members, and in religion.	Provide time to express and ventilate worries. Encourage family members to keep communication open. Keep reinforcing strengths. (Also apply nursing actions for objective 4.)

TABLE 2-8 (continued)

OBJECTIVES	NURSING ACTIONS

Diagnosis 2: Robert's Diabetes

Objectives: Short-term (after two visits)

OBJECTIVES	NURSING ACTIONS
1. Robert will have a positive relationship with community nurse, will be communicative and cooperative.	Use first visit to show interest in Robert's hobbies and daily activities. Try to get Robert to introduce nurse in his friendship circle. Walk with him downtown. Make him feel that he is appreciated as a person. Be nonjudgmental and express that nurse understands his behavior and his problems.
2. Robert will begin to change his behavior toward his mother, less anger and resistance.	On the way to town talk about mother and stress to Robert that she loves him and is worried and that she needs his help. Stress his strengths to him and abilities to help her.

Objectives: Intermediate (after 10 visits)

OBJECTIVES	NURSING ACTIONS
3. Satisfactory plan for managing diabetes regime. Injections will be given regularly. Diet in the home will follow diabetic guidelines. Urine will be tested every morning and recorded. Hygiene and foot care satisfactory without putting pressure on Mrs. Fox.	Include responsibilities for diabetes regime in objective 1–4. Initially visit the family several times for A.M. injection to relieve the daughter. Aim for the nurse doing one injection per week. Involve at least one more person besides daughter.
4. All family members involved have satisfactory awareness of diabetes and its maintenance.	Reinforce injection teaching to daughter and instruct a neighbor. Reinforce diet teaching to all members involved, Robert included. Include hints to make casseroles and other dishes usually brought in which are consistent with Robert's diet.
5. Robert is responsible and reliable about testing his urine. He will record it on a list and drop it off at the doctor's office once a week.	Teach Robert urine recording. Watch his testing procedure. Stress his reliability and give positive reinforcement for good performance. Instruct Mrs. Fox not to pressure him.

TABLE 2-8 (continued)

OBJECTIVES	NURSING ACTIONS
6. Robert is responsible for his own hygiene. He follows a schedule for showering and foot care according to his liking.	Discuss with Robert hygiene in relationship to his diabetes. Listen to his concerns and problems regarding following a schedule.
7. Family understands Robert's needs for independence and gives him opportunities to show his abilities. Family understands that setbacks and inconsistent behavior are to be expected.	Family discussion about meeting each other's needs and finding ways to help each other rather than forcing each other to perform. Aim at joint decision to take pressure off Robert. Warn that change will not be immediate, setbacks should be tolerated. List treatment aspects that have to be followed strictly: time of injection and meals. Encourage to apply pressure if Robert does not comply with these—Robert is told that these measures are vital if he wants to enjoy life. Other aspects: Showers, footbaths, sleeping in, and so on, will be treated with more leniency and Robert is given more control over them.
8. Robert will have a set of exercises for his legs to reduce deterioration due to neuropathy.	Get a PT evaluation and prescription of exercises. Practice them with Robert and help him set up a schedule.
9. Robert shows increased cooperation and less anger toward mother and sister.	See objective 2-7. Use sister's ability to communicate by pointing out that Robert responds to positive feedback and interest shown in who he is and what he can do. Help discuss problems still occurring over time.
Objective: Long-range (by termination)	
10. Robert's diabetes is under control. Some weight loss. Urines 1 + and no increase of insulin.	Should follow as a result of decreased dependence, a better sense of responsibility for self and the family, better communication. See also diagnoses 4 and 7.

TABLE 2-8 *(continued)*

OBJECTIVES	NURSING ACTIONS

Diagnosis 3: Mrs. Fox's Aging Process and Hypertensive Disorder

Objective: Short-term (after two visits)

OBJECTIVES	NURSING ACTIONS
1. Mrs. Fox will have visited the doctor for reevaluation of her condition and prescription of medication if necessary.	Monitor Mrs. Fox's blood pressure. Teach Mrs. Fox the serious consequences of untreated hypertension. Inform her about the nature of the disease and the medications with their side-effects. Encourage her to tolerate some side-effects as "the lesser evil."

Objective: Intermediate (after 10 visits)

OBJECTIVES	NURSING ACTIONS
2. Mrs. Fox will exhibit fewer symptoms of anxiety: better sleep, less frustration about losing control over self and Robert.	Keep monitoring BP. See objectives 1-3 and 1-4. Feeling of being able to control things reestablished through effective division of labor and changing of roles within the family.

Objective: Long-term (at termination)

OBJECTIVES	NURSING ACTIONS
3. The family will set up and discuss a plan with regard to Robert's care and support when Mrs. Fox will no longer be able to live independently and after her death.	Build this theme into regular family discussion. Slowly make them aware of the need to face the future. Mrs. Fox will be ready for it after she learns to cope with her present problems. Robert first needs to become more self-sufficient so that his real strengths can be built into the plan. There is possibility that Robert has a fear of institutionalization. Robert needs to participate and state what his ideal situation for the future should be.
4. Mrs. Fox uses religion as a comfort and source of strength.	Determine Mrs. Fox's involvement with the church and strength of religious belief. Use pastoral resources. Get Mrs. Fox involved in church activities for senior citizens.

TABLE 2-8 *(continued)*

OBJECTIVES	NURSING ACTIONS

Diagnosis 4: Communication Breakdown

Objectives: Short-term (after two visits)

See objective 1-2.

OBJECTIVES	NURSING ACTIONS
1. Mrs. Fox will have a beginning understanding of Robert's needs and related behavior. She will exert less pressure for compliance and will start to reward his progress.	Outline for Mrs. Fox Robert's needs and her own and explain Robert's frustrations based on his need for independence. Let Mrs. Fox determine some changes she may be willing to make. Encourage positive reinforcement of health-related behavior.

Objectives: Intermediate (after ten visits)

See objectives 2-7 and 2-9.

OBJECTIVES	NURSING ACTIONS
2. Robert's brother will act as mediator between Robert and family. He will influence Robert toward healthy behavior patterns.	Express to Robert's brother the family's need for his help. Explain the seriousness of Robert's condition and appeal to his concern for his brother. Discuss with him ways he could use his trust relationship with Robert to change his behavior—for example, interpret Mrs. Fox's controlling behavior as concern for Robert.
3. Robert's brother will have increased self-esteem based on his being needed. He will take on more responsibilities.	See objective 2-7.
4. Robert's sister will be content about her share of responsibilities and no longer needs to complain.	See objectives 1-4 and 2-7.

Objectives: Long-term (by termination)

OBJECTIVES	NURSING ACTIONS
5. Family develops own pattern of coping and dealing with problems on a basis of open communication and sharing between all members.	Act as role-model in family discussions. When family becomes skilled, withdraw for one session, later for more. Discuss with family how they handled problems without nurse and strengthen the belief in their own resources.

TABLE 2-8 (continued)

OBJECTIVES	NURSING ACTIONS
Diagnosis 5: Robert's Dependency *Objectives:* Short-term (after two visits) See objective 2-2. *Objectives:* Intermediate (after ten visits) See objectives 2-5 and 2-6.	
1. Robert will show concern for his diet, has an approximate idea of the kinds of foods included and the sizes of portions.	Include Robert in the diet teaching and reinforce signs of involvement. Test his understanding regularly and stress to him how helpful he can be to his mother.
2. Robert is included in the plan of labor division. The expectation for help is matched with his abilities.	See objective 1-4. Add tasks slowly as Robert finds satisfaction in completing his assignments. Make him feel good about accomplishments.
Objectives: Long-term (at termination)	
3. Robert likes to help in household. He volunteers for work in order to help mother and sister.	Continue positive reinforcement and make family members aware of the need for recognition of his efforts.
Diagnosis 6: Robert's Loss of Self-Esteem *Objectives:* Short-term (after two visits)	
1. Robert will exhibit more cooperative behavior based on his feeling of being better accepted.	See objectives 2-2 and 4-1.
Objectives: Intermediate (after ten visits)	
2. Robert will spend less time socializing with his friends. He will instead put more energy in his hobbies and responsibilities at home.	See objectives 1-4, 2-7, 5-2.

OBJECTIVES	NURSING ACTIONS
3. Robert will be involved in vocational testing and possibly training.	Refer Robert to community agency responsible for testing and job placement of the handicapped and mentally retarded. Act as liaison person between Robert and agency. Listen to Robert's concerns, fears, goals, and wishes. Make helping personnel of the agency aware of Robert's strengths and problems. Discuss with Robert aspects of change in daily routine—for example, getting up earlier, necessary when holding a job.
Objectives: Long-term (at termination)	
4. Robert will have gainful employment, possibly a job he could do at home.	Follow through with objective 6-3.
5. Robert will exhibit responsible behavior necessary to carry the job. He will control his emotional outbursts.	Include Robert's adjustment problems in family discussions. Follow through with objective 4-5.
6. Adjustments will be made by the family, and routine will be reorganized to accommodate change and still comply with diabetic routine. Transportation will be arranged for either through agency or community resources, if necessary.	Adjustments of task distribution within the family needs to be discussed and agreed upon.

OBJECTIVES	NURSING ACTIONS
Diagnosis 7: Noncompliance	
Objectives: Short-term (after two visits)	
See objective 2-2.	
Objectives: Intermediate (after ten visits)	
See objectives 5-1, 5-2, 6-2, 2-5, 2-6, 2-8.	
1. Robert will agree to and follow through with dental appointment and an eye checkup.	When Robert is ready, explain the importance of eye care in diabetes. Also let him see that it is needed for the search of employment. Gently persuade him to get dental repair done.
2. Robert will not accept food from his friends and will not visit the bar.	Arrange a talk with Robert's friends and stress the importance of not giving him food or drinks. Suggest to Robert that his diet outside the house is his responsibility and that the family needs his help. Discuss what kinds of diet he could eat when he visits and assess whether he would accept diet sodas in exchange for alcoholic drinks.
3. Robert will adjust his sleep and rest patterns by being active after breakfast—for example, doing his household chores.	When Robert is ready, discuss with him his sleep and rest pattern. Explain exercise in relation to insulin needs. Discuss compromises, such as a before-dinner nap if Robert insists on going to bed late. Let him express his concerns.
Objectives: Long term (at termination)	
4. Robert's eyesight is improved through corrective lenses.	Follow through on objective 7-1.
5. Robert's teeth are in good condition and Robert includes dental hygiene in his daily activity schedule.	Follow through on objective 7-1. Teach preventive dental care—brushing teeth effectively, or reinforce the dentist's teaching.

TABLE 2-8 (continued)

OBJECTIVES	NURSING ACTIONS
Diagnosis 8: Robert's Mistrust of People	
Objectives: Short-term (after two visits)	
See objective 2-1.	
Objective: Long-term (at termination)	
1. Robert feels fairly comfortable talking to helping people, such as employment agency personnel, dentist, eye doctor.	Accompany Robert to some agency visits and support him in social interaction with people he never met before.
2. Robert makes new friends in connection with his new work.	Observe Robert at work and encourage him to talk to others. Help him participate in small group discussions.
Diagnosis 9: Safety Problem	
Objectives: Intermediate (after ten visits)	
See objectives 1-4, 5-2, 4-3, 4-4.	
1. Family is aware of possible safety problems. Mrs. Fox is not left alone for long periods of time. Daughter and neighbors drop in regularly.	Teach family home safety and awareness of danger relative to old age, reduced visual acuity, forgetfulness and hearing loss. Remove hazards such as loose rugs. Install good lighting fixtures in hall, and night lights.
2. Procedure to follow in case of emergencies is established: Robert and Mrs. Fox know emergency numbers, fire extinguisher handy in kitchen—Robert knows how to use it, and so on.	Discuss emergency plan with family, go through a fire drill. Teach measures to follow in case of emergencies.

TABLE 2-9 ADDITIONAL NURSING ACTIONS, PRIMARY PREVENTION

All family members should be:

- Informed about the need for a balance between activities and rest.
- Urged to schedule activities to provide physical exercise and social and intellectual stimulation.
- Informed about and urged to use methods of relaxation.
- Made aware of their need for physical and emotional security and urged to undertake measures to provide it.
- Made aware of their need for self-esteem and asked to examine the adequacy of the sources of such esteem so they can make changes if needed or look for professional help.
- Made aware of their need for social support and asked to examine the adequacy of family and friends as support system in order to make changes if needed.
- Urged to examine their participation in social and religious activities and to determine its adequacy.
- Urged to examine the ways they cope with stress and the need for possible reduction of stress so they can seek professional help if needed.
- Urged to discuss ways in which changes can be made to reduce stress at work and at home.
- Made aware of the harmful effects of substance abuse on body and mind.
- Urged to get Mrs. Fox's son to get help for his alcohol problem and to provide him with support.
- Made aware of the importance of preventive medical, dental, and eye care and make provisions if needed.
- Urged to examine their medical insurance coverage to determine if it is adequate.
- Urged to become knowledgeable about VD and its prevention.
- Urged to practice good hygiene, cleanliness, and effective food preservation.
- Informed about the ways diseases are transmitted and how contamination can be prevented.

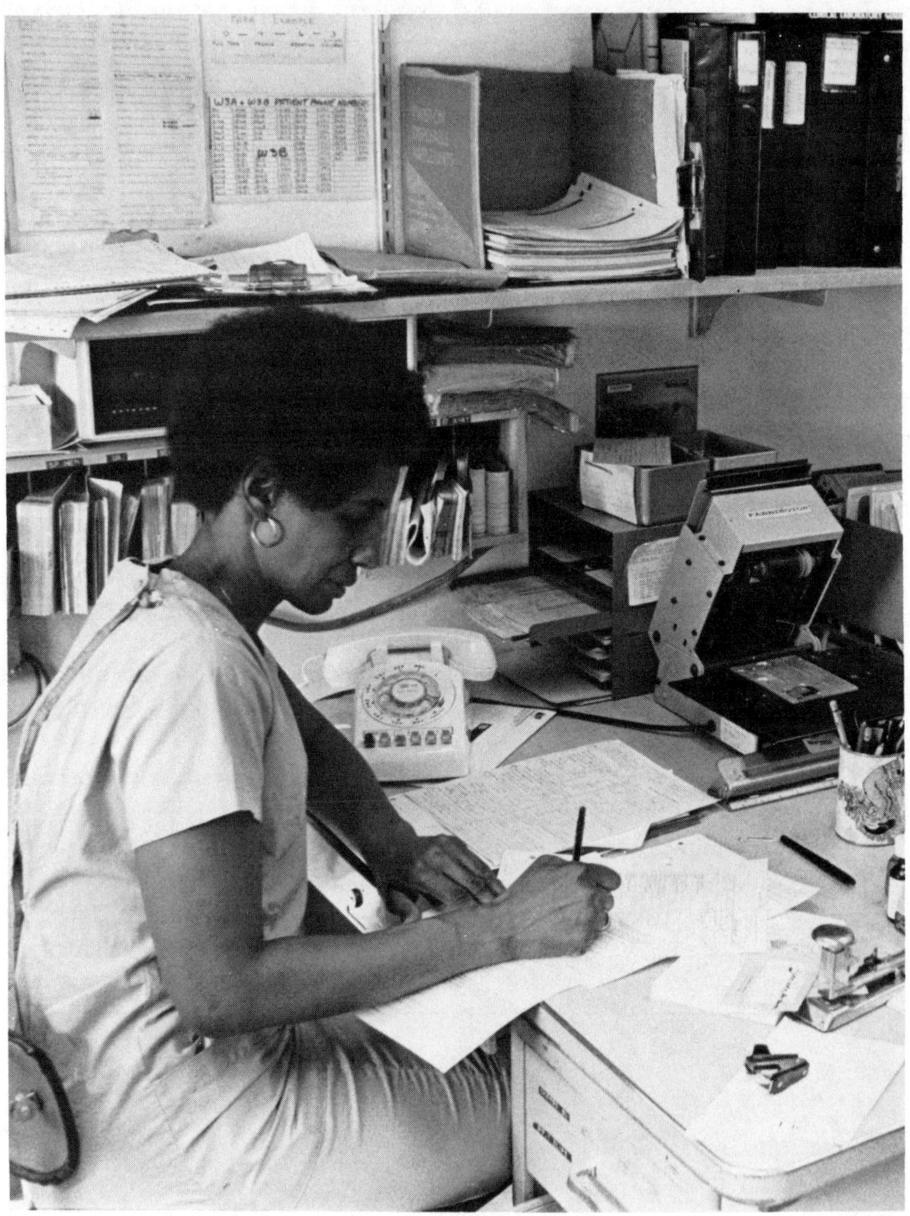

GEORGE FRYE

3

Implementation and Evaluation

The nurse has now reached the stage where the care plan can be put to a test. Even though this marks the start of the implementation phase, it does not end the other phases. In actuality, the implementation phase goes hand in hand with the evaluation phase and the assessment and planning phase. The implementation phase is an integration of all phases into one. While the nurse is executing the nursing actions, she should be continuously evaluating the family's responses to the interventions and observing with equal keenness any information to supplement the assessment. Just as one problem leads to many others within the family system, changes brought about by nursing interventions also lead to more changes. Thus, the conceptual framework of problem interaction cannot be considered to be a stable entity; it needs to be changed and updated on a regular basis. The nurse needs to be flexible and resourceful. Implementation should be a team effort and so should be evaluation. The family should be closely involved in the process, and their evaluation of nursing care should carry more weight than should the nurse's opinion, which is often less than totally objective. All possible community and family resources should be involved in the process, and the nurse should take on the role of a liaison person who helps the family adjust to the systems and policies of the community agencies involved or to the changes occurring within their own family system.

EVALUATION OF INDIVIDUAL AND FAMILY:
EVALUATION BY OBJECTIVES

Changes need to be recorded. If the care plan is based on problems (diagnoses), objectives, and corresponding nursing actions, the logical way to proceed is probably problem-oriented recording. That is, the nurse outlines the actions taken and then determines whether the objective was met and whether it needs to be further pursued or modified. Modified objectives are jotted down with newly proposed nursing actions.

An example using the Fox case will best illustrate the procedure; this is presented in Table 3-1. This kind of recording of interventions, coupled with modifications of actions based on ongoing evaluations, can be done for every objective in the care plan. The procedure is easiest to follow if each objective is allowed to occupy a separate page and ample space is made available for modifications. Objectives should then be ordered according to urgency, date, or projected accomplishment, which provides an overview of the effectiveness of interactions and also helps the nurse keep track of the time schedule. Accomplished objectives should be moved to the back of the record so that the most urgent ones are on top and visible.

EVALUATION OF INDIVIDUAL AND FAMILY:
EVALUATION OF THE PROBLEM LIST AND DIAGRAM

In addition to updating objectives and problem and strengths lists, the nurse should periodically evaluate the conceptual framework as well. He or she should look over the factors listed and cross out the problems that have been eliminated as well as their corresponding arrows on the conceptual framework. New problems or strengths should then be added to the list and the diagram. An adjusted diagram for Mrs. Fox would look like that shown in Figure 3-1; corrections are marked in parentheses.

Figure 3-1 shows that a few problems have been eliminated, but the ones that remain are fixed problems that are likely to get worse over time. Frustration, stress, and depression are still present even though the total lower half of the diagram of Figure 3-2 has been resolved through effective management of Robert's diabetes. Consequently, the emphasis of care must shift to utilization of modifiers rather than elimination of problems. Strengths such as religion, family support, and a workable plan to arrange for Robert's care after his mother's death (objective 3-3) now become of paramount importance. The community nurse needs to decide whether

TABLE 3-1. EVALUATION OF NURSING CARE FOR ROBERT FOX AND FAMILY

OBJECTIVE 2-1	ACTIONS	INTERVENTIONS	DATE
Robert will have a positive relationship with nurse, will be communicative and cooperative.	Use first visit to show interest in Robert's hobbies and daily activities. Try to get Robert to introduce nurse in his friendship circle. Walk with him downtown. Make him feel that he is appreciated as a person. Be nonjudgmental and express that I understand his behavior and problems.	Robert sitting on couch. No eye contact. Was either mute or volunteered one-word answers to questions. Changed approach: Presented myself and explained my role—help deal with some problems concerning the whole family, see to it that all people in the family could be healthier and happier. Asked Robert if he would help me. Responded by looking at me for the first time. Went on telling him about the good things I had heard about him. He seemed to listen closely, mumbled twice.	5/6
	Modified Actions Do not push Robert. Continue positive reinforcement and wait until he becomes verbal. Then proceed as above. Actions 5/9 completed. Robert now ready for actions of 5/6: Introduce nurse to friends. Walk downtown.	Robert looked at me and greeted me. He was dressed in spite of early hour. Commented to him my positive surprise and appreciation. He answered some of my questions concerning injections and insulin—knew about times the shots are given and rotating sites. Stated that he would be able to help me a lot to get things better. Asked him whether he would take me to the basement. He did. Became verbal, beaming facial expression. Explained his tools and models. I asked him many questions—he enjoyed being the expert.	5/9

Physical Needs	*Safety and Security Needs*	*Self-esteem and Esteem by Others*
Failing health; age	Forgetfulness	
Hypertension (controlled)	Problem with food safety (eliminated: Robert and sister are aware)	Frustration Stress
Weakness in left arm (constant)	Refusal to take medication	
	Possible accident proneness	Anger
Failing eyesight (worsening)	Dependency	Depression and lower self-esteem
Loss of strength and function		Decreased involvement in house and garden (not able to do more)
Tiredness (unchanged)		
Change in sleep pattern (now sleeps a lot)		
Lack of exercise (still minimal)		

FIGURE 3-1.   Problem diagram for Mrs. Fox evaluated.

she is prepared and confident enough to modify diagnoses 1 and 3 and their accompanying objectives and proceed with counseling based on new objectives. Many times, if resources are available, the client may prefer to proceed with a pastor or a mental health person. The community nurse should not exert any pressure, but leave it up to the client and family to decide.

As this example shows, if evaluation can be done before the nurse loses sight of the total interaction system, it will help avoid later problems or energy being wasted on unrealistic, unsolvable objectives. Changes affecting the conceptual framework equally affect the problem list and assessment data, as shown in Table 3-2. It is especially important to keep both of these tools current if more than one nurse is seeing the family.

As a result of these changes, diagnosis 3 should be modified. It should now read:

Inefficient coping of Mrs. Fox with loss of strength and function secondary to:
   • inability to gain confidence through religion;

Physical Needs	*Safety and Security Needs*	*Self-esteem and Esteem by Others*
Failing health; age	Forgetfulness	Frustration Stress
Weakness in left arm	Accident proneness	
Loss of strength and function	Dependency	Depression and low self-esteem
Tiredness		
Inability to exercise		
		Decreased ability to perform activities gaining self-esteem
	Security about matters being taken care of	
	Confidence through religion	
	Support through family	
	Esteem through accomplishments done in the past	

FIGURE 3-2.   Problem diagram for Robert Fox evaluated.

- *lack of security due to lack of satisfactory arrangement for Robert's care after her death;*
- *inability to look at her life as an accomplishment and as being complete;*
- *inability to fully accept family support as needed and deserved.*

EVALUATION OF INDIVIDUAL AND FAMILY: EVALUATION OF THE FAMILY'S OPTIMAL LEVEL OF FUNCTIONING

Table 3-3 outlines other evaluation procedures essential for the nursing process.

Evaluation done by objectives helps the nurse to understand changes and adapt to them as they happen. The procedure is necessary to eliminate, add, or modify objectives. The objectives express an ideal image of

TABLE 3-2. LIST OF PROBLEMS AND STRENGTHS FOR MRS. FOX REASSESSED

ASSESSMENT DATA	PREVIOUS ASSESSMENT				CURRENT ASSESSMENT			
	FP	AP	PP	S	FP	AP	PP	S
Age 92, failing health			x		x			
Widow of many years				x				x
Forgetfulness	x		x				x	
Hypertension	?	x			Controlled			
Refusal to take medications		x		x	Eliminated			
Thin, fragile appearance			x			x		
Dental prostheses			x				x	
Alertness, coordination, productive thinking				x				x
Weakness in left arm	x	?			x			
Depressed mood		x				x		
Activity and Rest Pattern								
Decreasing level of involvement in household and garden, increasing dependency	x	x			x			
Change in sleep pattern		x			Eliminated			
Lack of exercise		x			x			
Life Enjoyment and Satisfaction								
Able to handle household partially				x	Eliminated			
Now does very little in household					x			
Failing eyesight and memory			x		x		x	
Self-esteem derived through autonomy and independence		x				x		
Purpose for living—take care of Robert		x				x		
Delegated tasks					Nearly eliminated			
Inability to adapt to natural physical changes due to age		x				x		
Religious belief				x				x

TABLE 3-2 *(continued)*

ASSESSMENT DATA	PREVIOUS ASSESSMENT				CURRENT ASSESSMENT			
	FP	AP	PP	S	FP	AP	PP	S
Social Support System								
Mutual support within family				x				x
Daughter's willing to support family				x				x
Robert does not take part in supporting mother; affection not usually apparent		x				Resolved		
Trust relationship between brother and Robert		x		x				x
Mrs. Fox used to be center of family support, now daughter is taking over		x		x		x		x
Many friends and concerned people in town				x				x

the client's situation after all possible changes have been made and all fixed problems and strengths have been considered. In other words, it is the OLOF of the family. Short-term objectives are intermediate levels to be reached before the nurse strives for the optimum. The OLOF is based on a thorough understanding of the assessment data. However, since it is not possible to accumulate all possible data or to foresee every interaction between variables, the OLOF the nurse decides on is merely an educated guess. In every case, there are surprises that throw the plan off—either negative ones, as in the example of Mrs. Fox, or positive ones, as when progress is faster than anticipated. Either way the nurse needs to have a system for adjusting objectives and redirecting the care. It needs to be stressed again that a thorough and exact assessment and planning of care will greatly decrease the discrepancy between the assessed OLOF and the true OLOF of the family. The product will be less adjustment of the direction of care, less confusion for the client, better and faster results, savings in time and energy, and—above all—an impression on the client that the nurse is competent, efficient, and truly helpful.

TABLE 3-3. OTHER EVALUATION PROCEDURES

EVALUATION PROCEDURE	ASSESSMENT	CRITERIA
Individual Client/ Family Evaluation		
1. Determination of family's optimal level of functioning	Nursing assessment Discrepancy between previous state of health and present state of health Changes in level of functioning	Ideal state of health considering strengths and limitations of family. (Fluctuates with change of client problems)
2. Evaluation of nursing care	Nursing assessment	Objectives = operationalization of OLOF

Success of care is measured by the extent to which objectives are met. Evaluation leads to reassessment of client's state of health and modification of objectives.

EVALUATION PROCEDURE	ASSESSMENT	CRITERIA
Nursing Care Evaluative Research		
3. Project monitoring	Assessment of care implementation (audit of records, professional evaluation of nursing care of randomly selected cases)	Definition of nursing care Standards Procedures

Evaluation is a measurement of the discrepancy between assessment of actual care and standards for nursing care.

4. Impact evaluation	Assessment of pretreatment and posttreatment state of health/knowledge (sample of client population receiving identical care)	OLOF Defined objectives Client satisfaction

Evaluation is a measurement of *change* toward defined objectives and the extent of client satisfaction.

5. Cost-effectiveness study	Cost of service (time, manpower, materials, etc.)	Monetary gain for client (less hospitalization, employment, etc.) Monetary gain for community (reduction hospital beds, tax-income)

Evaluation is a measurement of the extent of monetary gain of the client and/or the community over the monetary investment involved in nursing care.

NURSING CARE EVALUATIVE RESEARCH

The more independently nurses function, the more crucial it is to evaluate the effectiveness of care. The purpose of such an evaluation is to establish credibility. The public needs to know that community health nurses handle problems efficiently and that the care they give is worth the money. In some small-scale, independent practices total nursing care has been made a reality; however, the formal evaluation procedure is generally neglected since it involves so much time, money, and training in research procedure.

What Blakely EJ (154, 1979) expresses in terms of research for community development holds true for nursing as well:

We need to know whether or not efforts have any of the effects they are purported to have. We need to know how these effects are brought about, and we need to know why they are not brought about if they are unsuccessful. Finally, we need to know something about the relationship between their costs and benefits so that we can make intelligent choices among alternatives.

Consequently, for nursing evaluation, research needs to answer the following questions:

- Is nursing care actually carried out as described in theory?
- Does nursing care actually result in the effect it claims to have on the clients' health status?
- Is nursing care cost-effective? Do the benefits warrant the money spent?

The first question could be answered by "project monitoring evaluation research" (Rossi PH et al., 122–157, 1979). In such a monitoring procedure, the first step is to define what nursing care actually is and list the standards and criteria that must be present. The second step is to audit records to determine whether care was performed according to the criteria. The researcher examines the assessment procedure and planning of care as outlined in the first part of this book as well as the implementation recorded by the nurse in charge of the family. Only if the standards of care are met and the researcher can comfortably state that the best possible nursing care is practiced in this agency or institution can the next step be undertaken. It is particularly important that the criteria of nursing care be specific and detailed enough that any other agency can adopt them and duplicate them. Different agencies working toward the same criteria by employing different methods may then be compared in order to test the efficiency of such methods. Such evaluation emphasizes the process.

The next step is "impact evaluation" (Rossi PM et al., 160–177), in which the effects of nursing care on the client family are examined and the changes toward the defined objectives are measured. Since the objectives cover all assessment areas, such change is not just of a physical nature but also social and psychological. To conduct an impact evaluation, data needs to be collected. In most agencies it is neither possible nor practical to conduct experimental research. This should not discourage the nurse from proceeding with the study using simpler methods such as nonrandomized samples.

In addition to the nurse's looking at how many and what kind of objectives have been met or how far the clients have progressed on the continuum of function, the clients should be asked their opinion about the same information. Client satisfaction is the best advertising power, and it tells the nurse that the service offered is what the consumer wants. If the service is congruent with the consumer's wishes, steps may be taken to get more consumers to want it by using publicity and advertising, political influence, grants for experimental nursing practices, and so on.

When that step is taken, it becomes crucial to conduct a cost-effectiveness study. If nurses want money for a project or services, they must learn to think in terms of money. Legislators are more impressed by figures that tell how many days of hospitalization were avoided through preventive care or how often institutionalization of an invalid was deterred through family guidance, or how many births were prevented by effective birth control, than they are by stories about nursing care improving clients' personal happiness. Thus, nurses have to learn to be aware of the necessity for conducting studies in order to have such data available.

Even if the need for data does not currently exist, nursing practice should be arranged so that data gets collected from the beginning until the end of a client's case. Records should be set up with the research aim in mind. The credibility of nursing care is often made most convincing by a demonstration of the long-term effects on the client family. Nurses of a weight-loss clinic, for instance, should show that their clients do not just lose weight but maintain it over time. Whenever feasible, a time study should be considered.

Such research efforts may be questioned as not being worth the time and money. However, I maintain that the benefits gained by a carefully constructed and organized study outweigh the efforts. Every sizable organization giving nursing care should seriously consider research. Even individuals should collect data on their clients and integrate it in a convincing manner so that they can show the public what has been achieved. Often a simple descriptive analysis is sufficient.

A second benefit of the research effort is the written or verbal feedback the care giver receives about client satisfaction. Throughout or at the end of the period of care, the nurse can use the shortcomings, misconceptions, and ineffective interventions revealed by such an evaluation as a way of learning and as a way of experiencing professional and personal growth.

REFERENCES

Blakely EJ: *Community Development Research: Concepts, Issues and Strategies.* New York, Human Sciences Press, 1979.

Rossi, PH, Freeman HE, Wright SR: *Evaluation: A Systematic Approach.* Beverly Hills, Calif, Sage Publications, 1979.

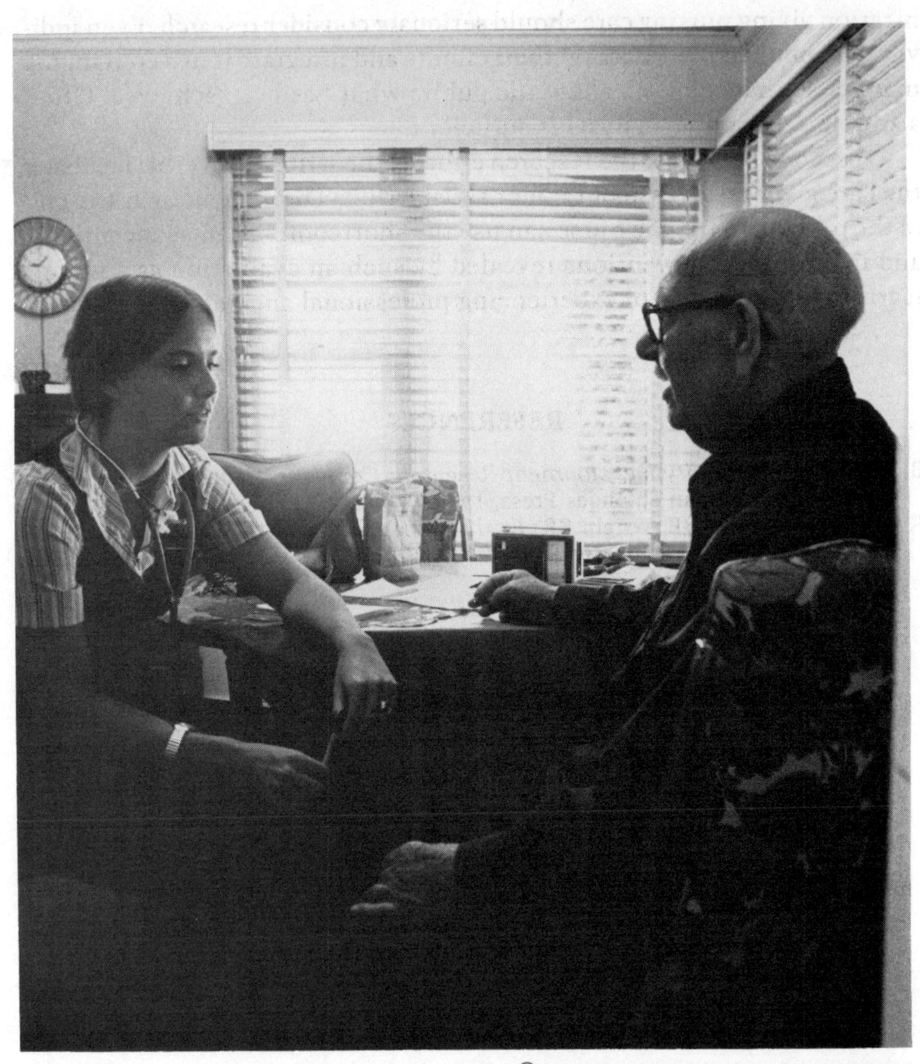

II

Patient Teaching for Self-Care

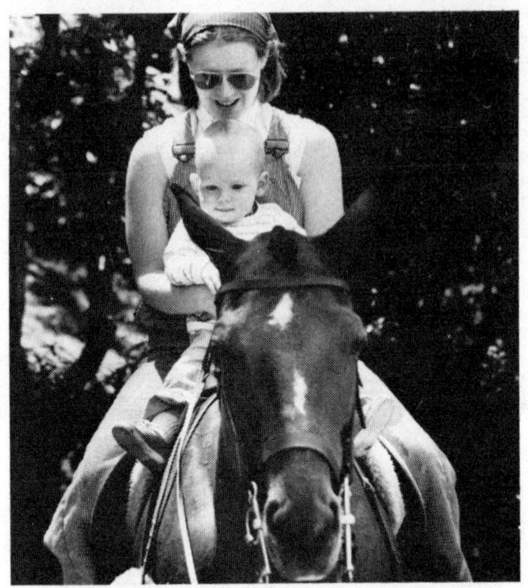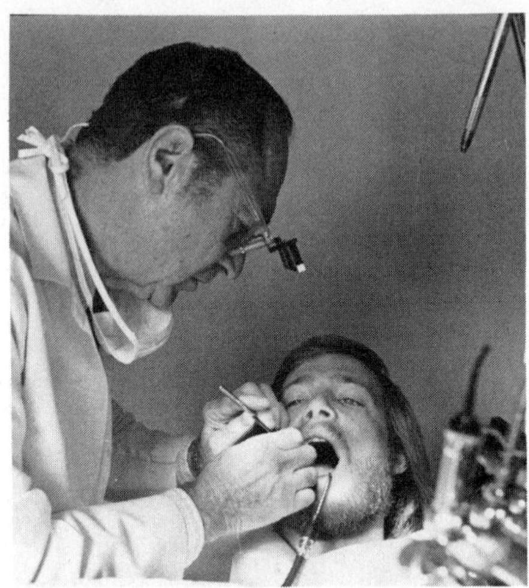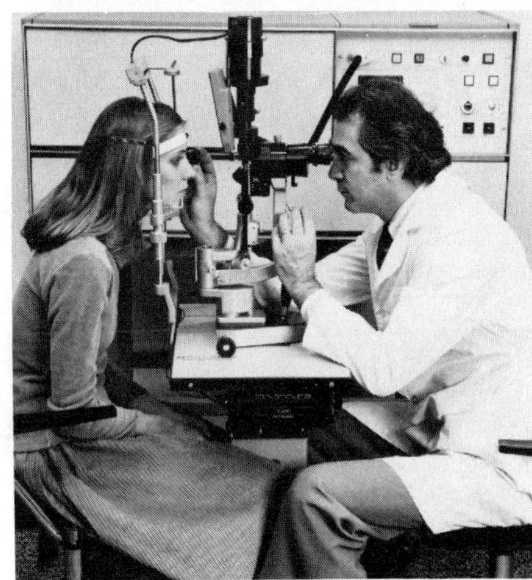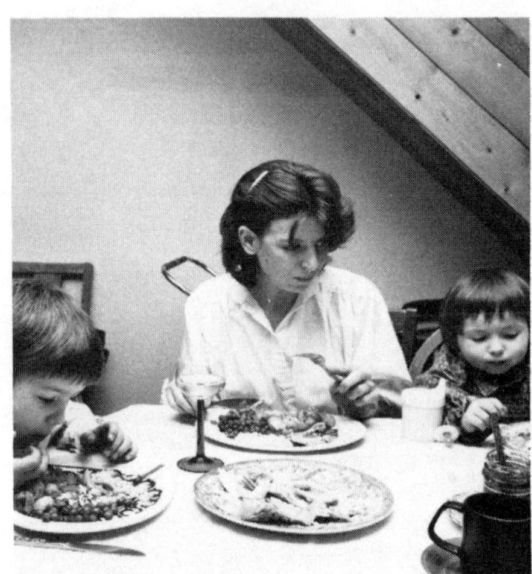

CLOCKWISE FROM TOP LEFT: ROSE SKYTTA, JEROBOAM, INC.; FREDRIK D. BODIN, STOCK, BOSTON; HAROLD S. CHAPMAN, JEROBOAM, INC.; HARRY WILKS, STOCK, BOSTON

4

Primary Prevention:
Teaching Healthy Families

If a client is initially seen as an emergency or for medical home care, several visits are primarily spent with crisis intervention and problem solving. Once the emergency is over, the nurse has a choice of discontinuing visits or of setting up a plan with the client to cover areas of primary prevention. Each client and family should be presented the option of a thorough nursing assessment and, depending on this assessment, one or more visits of preventive teaching. The option should not depend on the nurse's schedule or personal preference but should be entirely up to the client. The teaching plan should be discussed with the family and highly recommended if they show interest. Factors such as the client's schedule and financial situation must be respected, however, as well as the family's willingness to accept the teaching plan offered. If the client lacks motivation and does not fully approve of the teaching, no learning will take place.

Certain families may not be able to recognize the value of preventive teaching, even though the preliminary assessment suggests care is desperately needed. In such a case, the nurse may choose to spend several visits just socializing and building up trust in order to get the client to the point of wanting to listen (see Chapter 7).

If the client shows interest in primary care, the community nurse should present a plan of the areas to be covered which is based on an assessment. This chapter gives several tables that encompass the main areas of preventive teaching and offer suggestions for a lifestyle and preventive teaching program, which may serve as guidelines for the reader. The tables are geared to the person without physical problems or chronic disease—that is, the average person who needs to prevent illness by adopt-

105

ing a healthy way of living. Clients with short- or long-term medical and psychological problems will need modified care objectives, as will be discussed in Chapters 5 and 6.

The first step in setting up a teaching program for primary prevention is the assessment described in Chapter 1. Most of the information needed can be found in the assessment. However, the integration of the data is different. Using the example of the Fox family, primary prevention areas were initially assessed to find problems related to the key problems. Robert's hobbies or his daily walks to town were looked at because they are related to his noncompliance with the diabetic diet. The aim of the care was to solve the problems and get the family back to the status quo it had before the changes occurred. Primary prevention planning uses the same data after the main problems are solved or while they are still being treated. For the family without major health problems the assessment is primarily used for preventive teaching.

The assessment shows the nurse how knowledgeable the family is of each assessment area and where health practices are good or less than optimal. The initial questions the nurse asks are not concerned with problems but rather with how this family stands within the assessment areas in relation to optimal understanding and practice of preventive health.

The tools used by the nurse are a fairly stable set of objectives touching every assessment area. The objectives encompass all the knowledge the nurse thinks a client family should have about the assessment areas in order to be able to function optimally. In addition, the teaching program leads the family to apply such knowledge to their daily lives in order to reach their family's OLOF. Both teaching and implementation need to be adjusted according to individual family strengths, which make teaching possible, and barriers, such as handicaps, intellectual capacity, economic situation, educational background, and motivation. In the example of Robert Fox, the nurse would have to consider as one barrier Robert's mental capacity. Thus, any kind of diet teaching would have to be simply worded and employ visual aids. The nurse would need to realize that Robert learns better by doing than by listening to instructions, so that he would learn about diet best by weighing his hamburger or by selecting foods in the refrigerator and putting them together for a balanced meal. Because Robert showed no interest in self-care or diet teaching at the initial visit, it was clear that lecturing and teaching would have been ineffective and that a trust relationship had to be established with him first. Chapters 7 and 9 will discuss behavioral or cultural variables that influence the nurse-family relationship and the teaching process.

THE SELF-CARE TEACHING PROGRAM

The tables that follow in this chapter demonstrate a proposed teaching program for the family with the capacity and motivation for learning. When a family's circumstances are less than optimal, the nurse must be cautious about modifying this program. The teaching process should follow nine steps, as shown in Table 4-1.

TABLE 4-1. OUTLINE OF SELF-CARE TEACHING PROCEDURE

Step 1:   Assess client's motivation for learning.

Step 2:   Present outline of all the areas to be included in preventive teaching.

Step 3:   Contract with the family for an assessment and discussion of a treatment plan.

Step 4:   Make assessment. Include previous health practices within each area. (What objectives of Tables 4-2 to 4-7 are already met?)

Step 5:   Analyze all information collected and define areas of lack of knowledge and individual teaching needs.

Step 6:   Set up teaching plan covering all objectives not fully met by the family.

Step 7:   Project a time plan for teaching sessions.

Step 8:   Present teaching and time plans to the family and discuss them.

Step 9:   Adjust teaching plan according to the family's needs.

Let us assume that the community health nurse, after taking care of the Fox family's immediate problems, finds that Mrs. Fox's outlook on the future has improved and her depression diminished. The nurse is now ready to incorporate primary prevention teaching in visits over the next few weeks. The family, including Mrs. Fox's daughter and at times her older son, meets as a group once every two weeks in order to discuss progress and to listen to each other's concerns. The nurse judges that some preventive teaching can be accomplished if the family is willing to continue meeting for a few more sessions. It is clear the family members have made progress in sharing problems and concerns but that they still depend to a great extent on the nurse's presence. Hence, although the urgency of solving problems has diminished, further meetings are justified in order to prevent a communication breakdown caused by the nurse's premature withdrawal and to allow primary care teaching to take place.

During the next meeting the nurse presents the plan and watches carefully for signs of motivation. Mrs. Fox's daughter thinks it is a great idea, and, since she has found the biweekly meetings not too stressful for her, she feels she could continue with them, even though they require a bit too much of her time. Mrs. Fox seems to think she should not have to worry about these things any more at her age, but since she has enjoyed the meetings and found them helpful, she agrees to go along in order to make her daughter happy and perhaps benefit Robert. Robert is skeptical, but because the sessions have made him feel like an equal part of the family and his opinions have been valued, he shrugs his shoulders and says "okay."

Robert's brother is not present. The nurse urges the family to ask him to attend the meetings, since everyone is concerned about his health. Mrs. Fox states that if the sessions will enable him to accept substance-abuse treatment, she would really want to come. The nurse tactfully points out that the sessions are merely to help them learn about health, the effects of alcohol being only one of the topics, and that is how they should present the idea to Robert's brother; perhaps later he will at least begin to think about his drinking habit.

It is clear the motivation in the Fox family seems sufficient, but the nurse will have to make sure that the teaching is addressing *everyone's* needs and individual concerns, especially for those somewhat reluctant to go along. The nurse then presents the assessment and teaching areas and roughly outlines what will be covered. When someone expresses a special interest in an area or some concern, the nurse makes a note of it in order to include it in the teaching plan.

At the next session, the nurse makes an assessment of the diet and fluids for family members not previously assessed, asking questions similar to those in Table 4-2. As the family members discuss their interests in this area, the nurse clears up misconceptions, crosses out objectives they are knowledgeable about, and lists others to be included in the teaching plan.

It is important that some teaching is done while assessment data is being collected, since it stimulates interest and also serves as a justification for asking all these questions. If time permits, the nurse can also describe the areas in need of teaching and project the amount of time needed to cover them.

Usually one session is enough to assess and analyze one teaching area and arrive at an agreed-upon teaching plan. I prefer to treat every area separately, making an assessment and then teach within that area before proceeding to the next area, but some nurses prefer to do a complete assessment on all areas before presenting a teaching plan. Both methods can be effective: however, the complete assessment approach begs the patience of the family, since it must endure several sessions of questions without getting much feedback or learning new material. Thus, the family needs to be highly motivated with the latter approach.

In setting up a teaching plan, the nurse must give first priority to the family's concerns. The detailed plan, which is constructed after data on the areas of need has been collected, incorporates the nurse's scientific knowledge and practical experience. Problems beyond the nurse's scope should be handled by referring the family to community agencies, which the nurse should carefully explore for availability and services. The actual teaching process requires that the nurse have a good basic knowledge of teaching; some communication techniques and principles are described in Chapter 9. In addition, the nurse may make books, pamphlets, and audiovisual material available to the family.

The following tables in this chapter show how to construct a teaching plan on the basis of detailed assessment of each area.

DIET AND FLUIDS

In our society, the abundance of food has meant that the choice of foods is no longer a matter of availability but depends on each individual's judgment. Ideally, every person should know what foods are needed, how much, and why, but many people do not recognize the implications of poor food choice until they are struck with a chronic disease. Diet teaching is thus of major importance in preventive care.

In this area, many resources are available to nurses. There is a vast literature of diet plans, menus, and pamphlets on nutrition. Dieticians in hospitals and outpatient clinics are valuable information sources, especially if the client is known to the dietician owing to prior hospitalization or clinic visits. Some visiting agencies even employ their own dieticians; however, the teaching need is much greater than one person can handle, and so the dietician is best used as a resource person for nurses doing the actual primary care.

When teaching diet, the nurse should follow the steps listed in Table 4-1. Attempts to change diet habits in the direction of healthful nutrition patterns are subject to a high failure rate. Client motivation may be high, until they realize how many facets of their lifestyle are touched by this decision. It is hard to stick to a new diet regime since results are not immediate. Thus, nurses need to be cautious in assessing the client motivation and in making them aware of the pros and cons of diet changes.

TABLE 4-2. DIET AND FLUIDS

ASSESSMENT AREA	SAMPLE QUESTIONS	CLIENT OBJECTIVES	TEACHING AREAS
The four food groups	Have you ever heard of the four food groups? Do you remember what protein does for your body? What mineral and vitamin make milk such an important item in the diet? What does vitamin C do for your body? Vitamin C deficiency is called scurvy. Do you know the symptoms of this condition? How many servings of the bread group are recommended for lunch?	*At the end of the teaching sessions the client will:* • Name the types of foods listed in each group. • List the main nutrients, vitamins, and minerals in each food group. • Explain the function of nutrients, vitamins, and minerals in the body. • Outline the servings recommended for breakfast, lunch, and dinner.	The four food groups
Amounts of foods	Can you show me how big a hamburger you can eat for a serving of 2 ounces of meat? How big a banana makes up for one serving?	• State the daily caloric requirements for his height. • Estimate the size of servings of meat, vegetables, and fruit, or weigh and measure portions if greater precision is called for.	Number of servings required and size of such servings. Individualize according to height and age (use a chart)

	How many servings of each food group do you eat for dinner? Please make a list of the foods you had for yesterday's dinner.	• Recognize whether amounts eaten are comparable to recommended amounts.	
Fluids	What beverages do you usually drink? How much and how often do you drink liquids? Can you name few drinks that are high in sugar? Which drinks can you have in unlimited amounts without gaining weight? How much should a person drink in a day? What kind of nutritious drinks could you substitute for Kool-Aid?	• Name some drinks which are nutritious. • State that the ingredients in drinks usually accounting for a high number of calories are sugar or alcohol. • List drinks which do not add calories: water, coffee, tea. • State the daily recommended fluid requirements. • Examine whether change in fluid intake is needed.	Fluid requirement. Beverages as part of the diet to meet nutrition requirement.
Alcholic beverages	How often do you have an alcoholic drink? Do you drink with food? Do you drink socially? Do you drink when you are unhappy or upset? How many drinks do you usually take in one evening?	• State the effect of alcohol on the body. • Recognize emotional factors leading to drinking. • Explain the dynamics of addiction with continued excessive use of alcohol. • Examine own drinking pattern and assess whether change is needed.	Physical effects of alcohol abuse. Physical and emotional dependency with prolonged excessive consummation. Social and emotional factors of drinking.

TABLE 4-2 (continued)

ASSESSMENT AREA	SAMPLE QUESTIONS	CLIENT OBJECTIVES	TEACHING AREAS
Snacks	Do you eat between meals? What kind of snack food do you keep around? Do you get hungry in between meals? Are there some snacks you like which are good for your body? Why do you think high-sugar snacks are not recommended? What kind of changes can you think of that would least interfere with your lifestyle?	• Explain that snacking is not usually done because the body needs it but because of habit. • Define own snacking habits. • List nutritious snacks. • List high-calorie snacks with little nutritious value. • Examine whether change is needed.	Need for snacking. Nutritious snacks. High-calorie sugar snacks.
Frequency of meals	How many meals a day do you eat? Do you regularly skip breakfast? Do you eat your meals at a regular time or do you eat each time you are hungry? At what time of the day do you think your body needs food most?	• Recognize that the optimal pattern is three meals a day. • Recognize that skipping breakfast is an ineffective way of cutting calories. • Explain how frequent snacking leads to obesity. • State that breakfast is the most important meal of the day.	Importance of a regular meal plan. Control of excessive snacking. Importance of breakfast.
Likes and dislikes	Do you like milk? What foods do you eat instead of milk?	• Explain that most people can have a reasonably good diet if they follow their likes and dislikes within limits.	Incorporate likes into a healthy diet plan. Compromise family preferances.

	What are your likes in the meat, vegetable, and bread groups? Are you usually craving for sweets? Since you don't like carrots, what could you substitute for them?	• State that occasional sweets do no harm if the necessary other foods are eaten regularly. • Demonstrate the ability to substitute one food for another within the food groups.	Substitution of foods in the food groups with help of exchange list.
Eating habits	Do you eat slowly and chew your food well? Do you eat your meals in the kitchen or dining room? Do you skip meals? Are you rushed when eating or do you enjoy meals? Do you eat while you are doing other things? Do you feel tempted when walking by the refrigerator?	• List positive eating habits: eating regular meals, eating slowly, eating in one designated eating area only. • List negative eating habits: skipping meals, eating continuously, eating during activities (such as reading, TV watching), eating in many different places. • Explain physical effects of overeating. • Examine own habits and assess if change is needed.	Tips to avoid overeating and indigestion. Advantages of eating in a designated eating area only Importance of avoiding eating when doing other activities.
Emotional aspects of eating	Do you frequently eat with friends? Does food mean being sociable to you? Does eating make you feel better when you are sad or lonely? Is eating valued highly within your family? Does your family support your eating habits?	• State emotional reasons for wanting to eat. • Analyze the importance of food to self. • State why changes in eating habits are hard to make. • Explain cultural meaning food has for self.	Cultural aspects of food. Family tradition and eating Social aspects of food. Emotional gratification with food. Difficulties of diet changes

Unless clients decide that better health outweighs immediate gratification, their new diets are doomed to failure. Thus, they need a clear understanding of body function and nutrition.

The first key to success in teaching diet is *empathy*. A nurse must listen to the clients, explore their difficulties, and understand their diet problems in connection with work, family, problems, and other factors influencing eating habits. At times, it is better for the nurse to promote changes that are less than optimal but more likely to be accomplished by the client. A busy working mother, for instance, may resist getting up early to prepare breakfast but may be encouraged to take an apple to work to replace her regular doughnut during coffee break. Someone who gets much gratification from snacking may be better off changing the type of snack rather than giving up snacking altogether. Ideally, the change should be suggested by the clients themselves and the implications, good and bad, discussed with the nurse to prevent disappointment owing to results turning out less favorable than expected.

The second key to success, where nurses often fall short, is giving clients continuing support. The nurse may need to make several home visits, since a diet change must be permanently integrated into a client's lifestyle, a process that takes time and patience. Before discontinuing support, the nurse objectively needs to appraise the client's situation.

ACTIVITY AND REST PATTERNS

When working out a healthful activity-rest schedule for a family, a nurse must determine a balance of activities—physical and mental, work and leisure, solitary and social—to suit the clients' needs. Obviously, such a schedule will be very individualistic, since different persons find satisfaction in different activities.

How does a nurse decide whether a client's preferences are healthy or not? The key is *moderation*. This means that *each* of the assessment areas shown in Table 4-3 should be represented in the client's weekly activity schedule. Most people will prefer one or two areas, but a well-adjusted person will not exclude the remaining areas in favor of the preferred activity. A woman who favors arts and crafts in her free time should also set some time aside for physical activities. A man who finds competitive sports a source for self-esteem should also engage in some noncompetitive family activities or solitary occupations.

Besides looking for a balance among activities, the nurse should also look at how activities meet esteem needs. Work, for example, has different functions for different people. It may be a source of self-respect, because of the financial power or personal prestige it provides, or detract from self-respect, if the job does not fulfill expectations. For some people, the rewards of work are greater than mere status; work gives them a sense of achievement, pride, and respect. For such clients, leisure activities become less important than they do for clients who need them to make up for jobs of monotony or stress.

Within the activity-rest area there are eight need areas:

- Physical activity
- Mental activity
- Rest and sleep
- Self-respect and respect from others
- Togetherness
- Privacy
- Enjoyment
- Self-expression

When making an assessment, the nurse should look at each subarea with the client, exploring which needs are met by the activities the client regularly performs and which needs remain neglected. They can then explore other activities that might lead to the fulfillment of such needs.

Again, the teaching plan must rest on the client's motivation and willingness to change, but the nurse's empathy can help to make such change. The advantage of activity-rest teaching over diet teaching is that there are short-term, detectable results. Physical activities, for instance, provide an immediate sense of well-being, arts and crafts produce a finished product, and social activities may foster happiness and a sense of being liked by others. Resistance to change often derives from clients' extreme sense of duty, their working long hours, or their attempts to achieve perfection. On weekends, for example, clients may feel they have to mow the lawn, go shopping, or take their children out, so that their own needs and interests are neglected and they fail to have enjoyment in life. This leads us to the next area.

LIFE ENJOYMENT AND SATISFACTION

When assessing clients' emotional well-being, it is imperative that the nurse look first at their home situation, since this is where their basic needs should be met. Of course, some home situations are deplorable; a

TABLE 4-3. ACTIVITY AND REST PATTERNS

ASSESSMENT AREAS	SAMPLE QUESTIONS	CLIENT OBJECTIVES	TEACHING AREAS
		At the end of the teaching sessions the client will:	
Employment or daily occupation	How many hours a week do you work? Is your work physically strenuous or sedentary? Do you like your work?	• Realize effect of work on body and mind. • Explore satisfaction with work and possible need for change.	Meaning of work. Gaining self-esteem through work. Work as physical exercise.
Physical activity other than work	Are you involved in sports? Do you do any kind of exercise? Do you do your own house cleaning, cooking, and gardening? How do you keep physically active in winter? Do you have any ill effects when doing physical activities? Do you exercise with others or alone? Do you enjoy physical activity?	• Explain needs of body for physical activity. • State relationship of muscular, cardiac, pulmonary, gastrointestinal functions and exercise. • List effects of inactivity on body and mind. • Explore if change is needed. • Outline exercise program geared to individual needs, abilities, and limitations. • Follow healthful exercise program. • State cautionary measures when exercising.	Exercise and physiological functions. Exercise and mental functions. Effects of inactivity on body and mind. Combinations of exercise–fun, exercise–social functions, exercise–work. Limitations and precautions regarding exercise, related to age and physical ability.

Topic	Questions	Objectives	Content
Sleep and rest	How much sleep do you need? How much do you get? Do you have difficulties sleeping? Do you have problems falling asleep? Do you wake up in the middle of the night? Do you nap regularly? Do you have periods of rest when you work? How do you rest—lying down or sitting? Do you close your eyes?	• Explain the need of body for sleep and/or rest after physical activity and stress. • Outline ways to rest and relax after working or stress. • List possible measures of relaxation before sleeping. • Explore need for change. • Set up individual plan for resting and sleeping.	Importance of sleep with regard to functions of body and mind. Insomnia and measures to prevent and fight it. Relaxation techniques. Importance of resting while doing intellectual work. Ways to rest body and mind
Hobbies and activities other than sports and physical exercises	Do you have hobbies? What activities do you enjoy alone and with others? Do you find a sense of accomplishment in this activity? How much time each day do you spend with this activity? Does this activity serve for enjoyment and/or learning? Do members of your family appreciate your hobby?	• Explain the value of activities such as arts, craft, music, reading, and other pastime occupations. • Recognize the social value of pastime occupations. • State the individual value: sense of accomplishment and enjoyment of such activities. • Explore need for change. • Consider preferred activities and allow time for them on the daily schedule.	Function of hobbies and quiet activities as relaxation and rest. Stimulation of mental function. Creativity and self-expression. Fostering togetherness with games and other family activities.

very deprived family will be mainly concerned with meeting basic human needs, and so the nurse's attempt to teach any other health aspect will be futile. For these clients the first priority is crisis intervention—the involvement of other community agencies such as the health department, the housing commission, and the court in order to improve the living situation and provide food, linen, furniture, and supplies. With such families the nurse's role is one of a liaison person, a coordinator between different agencies and an advocate of client rights. A detailed family assessment may be vital for collection of evidence against a delinquent landlord or to mobilize community agencies. It may also be helpful in less drastic situations, since it may make the nurse aware of some problems not obvious at first sight. For instance, an elderly patient may not have the energy to get help for a plugged toilet, or the repair of a broken TV set might mean a little happier life for a client.

Table 4-4 presents questions that can be asked if additional information is needed beyond the family, home, or individual assessment. These questions are particularly useful if crisis intervention has previously been necessary. When the nurse begins preventive teaching, he or she should again ask questions about living conditions in order to reassess the situation. For instance, the family may have lived under less than optimal conditions before a crisis occurred and will consider this standard as normal. In this instance, the teaching plan has the aim of making the home a more hospitable place, helping family members be aware of safety hazards, and showing them how to plan ahead in providing food, clothing and future security. The teaching plan involves not only the client family's strengths and resources but community resources as well; the nurse should help the family members mobilize these resources so that they will stop feeling victimized and start to believe in their own power to influence daily events.

Following Maslow's hierarchy of needs, as listed in Table 4-4, safety is the next need to be considered after physical needs. During the home assessment, as the nurse explores with the client problems of the home's furnishing, sanitation, and so on, any problems with safety factors will become evident. The nurse can find out from the client what aspects they have already thought of and can help motivate the family by showing appreciation for their independent efforts and by gently suggesting improvements. Of course, motivation depends in part on the family's readiness; suggesting ways to child-proof a house after the first baby has been born will probably be accepted more readily than will suggestions for safer furniture for an old person emotionally attached to a rickety rocking chair.

Emotional safety is the next need to consider. Here empathy is important. If the nurse uses empathy with the elderly person above, giving her a chance to express herself and reveal the priority of her needs, she may demonstrate to the nurse that the idea of safe furniture actually threatens her—that she feels she would lose part of her home, her feeling of being safe in her surroundings. This will signal the nurse that in this case emotional safety stands in direct opposition to physical safety; however, only the client can weigh the two and make the best choice after being helped to consider all consequences.

The next need, financial security, might seem essential to emotional security, but it is not always. A well-to-do person may feel emotionally insecure worrying about impending tragedies, and someone without a stable income may feel quite emotionally secure owing to firm religious belief and family support. Emotional security is a state of minimal anxiety in which people rely on their own resources, or those of friends or a Supreme Being, and think positively about their future.

Self-esteem, the next need, is recognized as being a necessary component from childhood on for emotional security (Aguilera and Messick, 100, 1974). People have to have trust in themselves and feel that they have the power to handle their lives. People who are at the mercy of influential forces do not know what to expect next and so experience high anxiety. In assessing a client's emotional well-being, a nurse must be aware of the direct relationship between self-esteem and happiness. A positive self-concept not only fosters emotional security but also allows people the liberty to explore and gives them the strength to overcome temporary failures and misfortune (Pasquali et al, 76, 1981). People with negative self-concepts or low self-esteem, on the other hand, do not enjoy full happiness. They feel anxious, depressed, and socially isolated and so exhibit insufficient emotional security. The best way for a nurse to assess clients' ability to enjoy life is simply to listen and show concern for their problems. The extent of these problems will soon become evident. At times the mere presence of the nurse is comforting to clients; they feel more worthy because someone seems to care about them.

Even if the community health nurse does not feel equipped to handle complex mental health problems such as a lack of self-esteem, inability to make decisions, helplessness, and dependency, he or she can help clients gain strength and courage by listening empathetically. The nurse can help

TABLE 4-4. LIFE ENJOYMENT AND SATISFACTION

ASSESSMENT AREAS	SAMPLE QUESTIONS	CLIENT OBJECTIVES	TEACHING AREAS
Maslow's hierarchy of needs		*At the end of the teaching sessions, the client will:*	

Physical needs
  Food
  Drink
  Clothing
  Shelter
  Sex
	Can you manage to get enough food with food stamps?
	
	Do the children get hot lunch in school?
	
	Do you have friends who hand you down clothes for the children?
	
	Can you buy enough oil to heat your place in winter?
	
	Does your toilet work properly?
	
	What do you use to control roaches?
	
	Does your landlord know you have rats in the apartment?
	
	Do all your children have a bed of their own?
	
	Do you have enough sheets and towels?
	
	Is your relationship with your husband a happy one?
		• Have a satisfactory provision of resources to meet physical needs.
		
		• Live in a health-promoting environment: satisfactory sanitary conditions, electricity, water, heat, rodent control, insect control, and with sufficient space, furniture, and supplies.
		
		• State the principles of hygiene and relationship of cleanliness and health.
		
		• Share problems of sexual nature which interfere with enjoyment of life. (Reluctance to do so needs to be respected.)
		
		• Accept a referral to mental health or sexual counseling if emotional problems are extensive.
			Available community agencies.
			
			Principles of hygiene and cleanliness.
			
			Importance of good education.
			
			Relationship between health and living conditions.

Security needs Physical safety	Are your children able to stay by themselves when you leave the house? Does your family know what to do in case of fire? Do you have smoke detectors? Where do you keep your cleansers and medications? Have you ever thought of attaching this rug to the floor? Where is your baby usually when you cook dinner? Does your baby like to pull electric cords? Do you have a nightlight in the hall?	• List principles of safety. • List safety precautions at home and at work. • Explain recreational safety. • Assess if change is needed at home or outside the home. • Make the change.	Safety precautions at home: electric appliances, electric outlets, heat, cooking with gas or electricity, poisonous substances, furniture safety lighting, loose rugs, stairs. Industrial safety, outdoor and recreational safety. Fire precaution and disaster training.
Emotional security (What provides a sense of security—the town, place of living, belongings, family, religion? It is anything a person feels attached to and represents part of that person's integrity.)	How long have you lived in this place? Did you grow up in this town? Does your family visit often? Is your job situation stable? Do you belong to a church? How much does religion mean to you?	• Feel secure and comfortable in his or her surroundings. • Feel confident with self and others. • Understand relationship of happiness and emotional security.	Cannot be taught.

TABLE 4-4 *(continued)*

ASSESSMENT AREA	SAMPLE QUESTIONS	CLIENT OBJECTIVES	TEACHING AREAS
Financial security	Are you likely to lose your job in the near future? What is your chance of finding a new job? Did you apply for Medicaid or AFDC? Do you have contact with a social worker? Do you have difficulties meeting your financial commitments?	• Explore reality of threats to financial situation. • Start to make financial plans for the future in an attempt to avoid crises. • Seek assistance if unable to manage finances.	Credit counseling and other community resources if necessary.
Need for self-esteem and esteem by others	Do you like your work? Do you feel good about your life and your accomplishments? What was the greatest achievement in your life? Tell me three positive things about yourself. What activity makes you feel worthwhile? Do you feel that other people appreciate your effort? How does getting older affect you? What goals have you set for yourself?	• Describe the relationship of liking self and being liked by others. • Describe the relationship between achievement and happiness, failure and loss of self-esteem. • Outline how a sense of approval, and willingness to explore new interests and to work for others, influence self-confidence. • Set reasonable goals and work toward their achievement. • Recognize strengths and weaknesses in self.	Relationship between life enjoyment and satisfaction and self-esteem, body image purpose in life, goal setting achievement, sense of worth. Relationship between unhappiness and failure, depression, loss of self-esteem, insecurity, social isolation.

clients decide whether specialized professional treatment is needed and weigh the clients' strengths and weaknesses to determine with them whether their resources are sufficient to cope effectively and to regain satisfaction in life.

SOCIAL SUPPORT SYSTEMS

Social support systems (see Table 4-5) are an integral part of emotional security. A person needs to feel part of a family or a circle of friends. Lack of meaningful interpersonal relationship leads to loneliness.

In assessing this area, the nurse will be come aware of many differences. Some persons have a strong need to be among people, to be involved in social activities, and to feel liked by many. Others prefer to be alone and only occasionally seek company. A nurse may be eager to prescribe social activities for single persons, but these clients may not feel a great need for socialization. Others may feel more lonely among many people than by themselves; thus, a nurse cannot assume that people will be happy just by being among other people. While this variety in the need for social interaction makes it difficult for a nurse to assess whether clients' social systems are satisfactory or need change, the clearest indicator is loneliness. When they are lonely, clients are acutely aware of it and will express unhappiness about the lack of intimate friends or people who care.

Loneliness is a feeling from within, but it is related to self-esteem and esteem by others. Lonely people feel not liked by or worthy of others, and they keep away from others. Thus, they remain socially isolated even though they may long for companionship. In addition, they may be angry about people not caring for them, but make every effort to discourage such caring (Haber et al., 309, 1978).

There is no simple solution for happiness in this area. It demands careful listening on the part of the nurse and understanding of social isolation as a symptom of other emotional problems. Some clients may benefit from concern and empathy; others may need measures such as a goal to live for, someone or something to care for (even a pet), or a worthwhile task to pursue rather than social clubs and parties. Still others may have problems beyond the nurse's realm and may need to be referred to a mental health agency.

TABLE 4-5. SOCIAL SUPPORT SYSTEM

ASSESSMENT AREAS	SAMPLE QUESTIONS	CLIENT OBJECTIVES	TEACHING AREAS
		At the end of the teaching sessions, the client will:	
Family support	Who lives with you in your home? Do your sons and daughters visit you often? How far away do your brothers and sisters live? Are your parents still living?	• Recognize the importance of maintaining ties with family members or friends he or she feels close to.	Humans as part of a family a social system. Dependency on social interaction.
Friendship circle	Do you have some close friends? Who cares for you when you are ill? To whom do you go when you have a problem? Are all of your friends back in your hometown? How do you win new friends when you move to a new town? What person do you feel closest to?	• State the value of true friendship, especially in times of stress and need. • Outline steps to take in order to win someone's friendship. • Apply these steps.	Making friends by unselfish caring, getting involved, trusting others, helping and accepting help from others.

Social circle	Do you belong to any clubs? Do you participate in community activities? Are you active in church? Do you entertain in your home frequently? Do you go to parties? Do you have a good relationship with people at work? Do you spend lunchtime with your associates at work? Do you discuss everyday problems with others?	• State that he or she needs involvement with people, companionship and sharing. • Explore need for change. • Show willingness to explore possibilities for social involvement and pursue them.	Need for social interaction. Community resources and possibilities for involvement.
Religious support	How much does religion mean to you? Do you believe in God's power to guide you?	• Explore religion as possible source of strength and guidance.	Meaning of religion to humans.

STRESS AND STRESS PREVENTION

One reason for people's unhappiness, helplessness, and resignation is their inability to cope with stress. Stress seems to be a major factor in psychosomatic disease, and major physical conditions such as cardiac disease and peptic ulcer are accelerated by it.

Research on stress started after the publication of Selye's first book (Selye, 1956), and the knowledge base is getting larger. Selye sees stress as the effects of threatening or dangerous agents on the body, which is continuously adapting with the help of physiological mechanisms. Once these mechanisms are overtaxed, the nervous system, hormones, and endocrine glands are affected and eventually there is damage to the organ systems as well. Adaptation to stress depends on the individual's ability to maintain a balance within the internal physiological processes.

Stress is a natural phenomenon, and the threatening agents or stressors are of three different dimensions—external, internal, or psychosocial (Haber et al., 409–414, 1978). Every organism is equipped to adapt to external stressors, such as cold, humidity, infection, heat exposure, so long as they stay within limits. The body can be trained to adapt more effectively by repeatedly exposing it to stressors—for example, as has been done in space training for astronauts. However, today's society has created more external stressors, such as environmental pollutants, radiation, and noise, some of which may overtax human systems of adaptation.

Internal stressors are any agents that throw the internal physiological environment out of balance. Examples are hunger, endocrine or organ dysfunction, or sensory overload such as shell shock. The effect of such stressors is influenced by hereditary factors, which determine the vulnerability of certain organs or transmission of genetic disease. Internal stressors also determine to a certain degree how people perceive their world. According to Wolff (1953), this perception is based on early childhood experience; the stress response is reactivated when similar occurrences happen in later life.

Psychosocial stressors are those occurrences in daily life which cause a response of anxiety, anger, or frustration. Levi's (Chap. 3, 1972) research has shown that not only negative arousal but positive responses of excitement and elation may be stressful, since they may result in a depressive reaction after the excitement is over, as is often seen after Christmas or on Mondays after a good weekend. Psychosocial stressors are found in situations in which people interact; the most intense experiences happen within the family and at work, the amount of intensity depending on the emotional investment a person has made in another person. Whether occurrences are treated as stressful or not also depends on individual value systems, family cultural background, and other natural crises such as maturational changes. In addition, the rate of social change has been found to be closely related to adaptation to stress. Finally, research has found a significant relationship between change-related stress and the occurrence of physical disease. Holmes and Rahe (1967) developed a Social Readjustment Rating Scale, which they claim predicts the likelihood of onset of physical symptoms based on changes in life circumstances. The scale is easy to use and can be helpful to the community health nurse in stress assessment.

For the community health nurse the aim of teaching should be to give the family a clear understanding of stress, both avoidable and unavoidable, and to show the individual members how to be alert to the many warning symptoms of stress: fatigue, irritability, difficulty concentrating, insomnia, nausea, headaches, high blood pressure, diarrhea or constipation, feelings of undefined anxiety, powerlessness, depression, and others. The original assessment will indicate the main areas of stress, and clients will add others during the course of teaching. The nurse should also help individuals look at how they cope with stress, using examples of effective coping in the past to enable them to find ways to handle current crises. With the nurse, the family needs to decide on what changes need to be made, devise a plan for eliminating avoidable stressors or modifying unavoidable ones, and develop resources for coping. Strengths pointed out in the original assessment will be incorporated by the nurse in a plan for stress modification. In teaching, the nurse has many resources available: diet teaching, tips to parents regarding child development, relaxation methods to overcome insomnia, tension release exercises, and many others. In cases where stress modification goes beyond the nurse's skills, referrals may be necessary to counselors specializing in marital, sexual, or severe behavior problems. Stress is such a complex area that Table 4-6 can in no way encompass all the facets of it. The nurse will need to employ creativity in adjusting the teaching program to the family's individual needs.

PREVENTIVE MEDICAL, DENTAL, AND EYE CARE

This assessment area has traditionally been a high priority area in public health nursing, the main aim of which has been communicable-disease control. As Table 4-7 shows, the assessment consists of a set of concise questions, many of which require only a short answer. Examples are "Who is your family doctor?" and "How long ago did you have a TB

TABLE 4-6. STRESS AND STRESS PREVENTION

ASSESSMENT AREAS	SAMPLE QUESTIONS	CLIENT OBJECTIVES	TEACHING AREAS
		At the end of the teaching sessions, the client will:	
Knowledge about stress, its nature and physiological effect on the body	Have you ever heard or read about stress? What do you know about the body's reactions to stress?	• Understand and state that stress is the wear and tear on the body over time. • Explain that the body is in a dynamic state of equilibrium, continuously adjusting to stress with the help of physiological mechanisms.	Nature of stress and physiological effects.
Knowledge about types of stressors and their relationship to each other	What is your understanding of a stressor? Have you ever realized that a stressor may be beneficial to us? What kind of external, internal, psychosocial stressors can you see that influence your life? How do you think heredity may affect the stress equilibrium?	• State that there are three different kinds of stressors, all interacting with each relationship to other. • Give examples of external stressors, internal stressors, psychosocial stressors. • Explain the action of the above stressors. • Understand and discuss influencing factors—for example, heredity, culture, early childhood experiences, and perception.	Classification of stressors. Examples and action of such stressors. Beneficial action of stressors. Factors influencing stressors and their effect on each other and on stress.

	Do you think that people of all cultures react to the same stressor? Do you believe that heredity and childhood experiences have something to do with the way you look at the world?		
Knowledge about warning symptoms or signals that stress is present	How do you know when you are under stress?	• List the warning symptoms of excessive stress • Outline symptoms he or she has felt in the past or still feels.	Warning symptoms of stress. Excessive stress and its physical illness.
Presence of such warning signals in the present and past	After something unpleasant happened to you, have you felt very tired, or unable to sleep?	• State present and past situations leading to such symptoms. • Mention examples of stress-related illnesses as seen with friends or relatives.	Stress-related illnesses.
Stress-related situations in client's life	After a hard day's work, at times are you irritable and short-tempered? Have you ever felt that you were unable to relax or let go? Do you know anyone who has an illness brought on by too much stress? What kind of stress do you encounter outside and inside the family?	• Express awareness of own stress-related situations.	Explore with client stressors of all kinds.

TABLE 4-6 *(continued)*

ASSESSMENT AREA	SAMPLE QUESTIONS	CLIENT OBJECTIVES	TEACHING AREAS
Coping mechanisms in the past and the present. Stress in the family. Stress-related to maturational stages.	Have you had similar stress situations in the past? Have you learned from such experiences? Which ways of dealing with stress that you learned in the past could you use now? Do you think diet may have something to do with your lack of energy? Since you cannot avoid the stress of getting up at night for the baby's bottle, can you see any other ways of getting the rest you need? Are these changes possible and realistic for you to carry out?	• Outline the main source of stress. • Describe how he or she has coped with similar stress in the past. • Recognize and discuss family stress affecting all members. • Mention examples of maturational stress in the family. • Together with the nurse, set up a plan to modify stress. • Decide what changes he or she wants to make. • Follow the stress reduction plan.	Explore coping mechanisms and feasibility for present stressors. Stress reduction tools. Related areas leading to stress—for example, diet or exercise. Unavoidable stress versus avoidable stress. Planning structured approach to reduce stress.

test?" Clients usually expect these questions when visited by public health nurses and so are mentally prepared to answer them. Anything beyond that, however, may be quite surprising to them.

Although these simple questions should not be neglected by the community health nurse, they should be viewed as questions designed to open up broader discussions about the areas of preventive health and clients' health practices. After the clients name the family physician, for instance, the nurse may lead the conversation toward the health practices the physician recommends, such as immunizations, or suggestions for emergencies, or his or her ideas about routine use of nonprescription medicines such as aspirin or cough syrup. After ascertaining the family's awareness in these areas, the nurse can expand on what measures should be taken and why, such as temperature taking, distinguishing chicken-pox from a poison-ivy rash, or guidelines for keeping children home from school when they have diarrhea or upset stomachs.

When clients mention their dentist's name, the nurse may discuss preventive dental practices, including brushing, flossing, and diet. Questions about the birth-control methods used by the women in the family can lead to further questions and, in future nurse visits, to literature about birth control methods, sterilization, and so on, and their advantages and disadvantages. If the family shows interest, the nurse may also discuss venereal disease; this can be done in such a way that it involves no embarrassment or fears that the nurse suspects something. VD teaching is especially important if the family has teenagers. Families are often willing to listen to a nurse talk about sex education in the privacy of their home even if they oppose such education in schools. (See Chapter 9.)

The possibilities for teaching about medical, dental, and eye care are almost unlimited. Table 4-7 outlines only the most basic aspects. Some families may have excellent knowledge of health practices in these areas and require only additional literature and book references. Other families may be less literate and need more attention by the nurse. Many people get some ideas from the news media about preventive health practices; television commercials may urge them to quit smoking or to be aware of warning cancer signs. However, they may need the nurse to demonstrate a breast exam, tell them what a pap test feels like, to tell them how health information applies to their lives and what choices they have. Thus, a creative teaching program should be based on clients' understanding of preventive care, level of education, willingness to learn, and their needs with regard to their present health practices. The success of the teaching plan, however, is related to the nurse's skills at listening, teaching methods used, creativity of the approach, and ability to communicate.

TABLE 4-7. PREVENTIVE MEDICAL, DENTAL, AND EYE CARE

ASSESSMENT AREAS	SAMPLE QUESTIONS	CLIENT OBJECTIVES	TEACHING AREAS
		At the end of the teaching sessions, the client will:	
Medical care providers: regular emergencies specialists	Who is your family doctor? Do you have a pediatrician or do you use a clinic? Where do you go if your child runs a sudden high fever? Can you call your doctor for advice?	• Name the source(s) of regular health care for the family. • Outline a plan to follow in case of emergency: emergency phone number, doctor's office or clinic, night emergency station.	Importance of medical preventive care. Advantage of seeing a physician or medical facility regularly. Emergency medical plan: whom to call and where to go.
Dental and eye care providers	Do you have a dentist? Has your child ever visited a dentist? Who prescribed your glasses? Did you ever have an eye exam?	• Have a private dentist or will be registered at a dental clinic. • Name an eye doctor (preferably an ophthalmologist) and plan to visit him or her regularly.	Preventive dental care for better health and to save money. Preventive eye care: early detection of glaucoma, vision important for children learning and for accident prevention for the elderly.
Frequency of preventive health care visits	Have you recently visited your doctor? How often do you have a physical exam done?	• State the importance and reason for physical exams and chest X rays. • Make plans for a doctor's visit if needed.	

	Do you take your child to the clinic for checkups? How often do you see the dental hygienist? When did you have your last eye exam?	• State advantages of preventive dental care. • Explain need for regular eye exam. • Make an eye care appointment if necessary.	
Financial situation	Do you have medical-dental insurance? Does your insurance cover eye exams and glasses? Do you have Medicaid coverage? Do you have problems paying your medical and dental bills?	• Be aware of possibilities for financial help. • Make use of community resources if needed. • Accept a referral to a community agency if needed.	Facilities for low-cost and free medical and dental care Resources for financing dental and eye care. Assistance with application for Medicaid or referral to social worker if needed.
Birth control and venereal disease prevention	Do you practice any kind of birth control? Do you plan to have any more children? Do you consider contraceptives for your teenaged daughter? Do you feel emotionally ready for a tubal litigation? Have you and your husband discussed his plans for a vasectomy?	• Explain the different methods of birth control, action, and application. • State their use, indication, contraindication, and risk. • Outline sterilization procedures. • Be able to make a wise choice of birth control method based on all related factors. • Be free to express worries about VD and own sexual practices.	Methods of birth control, pros and cons. Sterilization procedures if applicable. Physiology of reproduction necessary to understand birth control. VD symptoms, implications, treatment. VD prevention. Community facilities for VD and birth control.

TABLE 4-7 *(continued)*

ASSESSMENT AREA	SAMPLE QUESTIONS	CLIENT OBJECTIVES	TEACHING AREAS
	Did you ever contract VD? Do you know how to recognize gonorrhea? What can you do to reduce the risk of contracting VD? Where would you go if you had VD symptoms or if your friend did? Are you aware of what happens if you get VD several times in a row? Do you know what complications you can get with gonorrhea?	• Explain symptoms and procedure to follow if they should occur. • Exert caution in sexual practices. • Express willingness to seek treatment if symptoms should occur.	Ways of spreading VD and need for tracing contacts. Danger of reinfection or inadequate treatment. Active and passive immunity. Diseases and their danger of permanent damage or death Methods of immunization and possible reactions.
Communicable disease prevention	Are your children's required immunizations up to date? How long ago did you have a TB test? Do you know what a positive TB test reaction looks like? Have you had a preventive tetanus shot lately? What diseases are preventable with immunization?	• Express awareness of necessity for immunization based on danger of contracting the disease and potential hazard to others. • Be willing to follow immunization regime for children and self. • Verbalize the necessity for regular TB tests or chest X rays and make the arrangement for one or the other if necessary.	Implications of TB and methods of control. Food poisoning and how to prevent it: food handling, refrigeration, defrosting, cleanliness. Correct canning procedures

	Is your refrigerator in working order? Do you do your own canning?	• Exercise safe methods of handling food and refrigeration. • Be aware of dangers of incorrect canning procedures. • State the importance of handwashing and good sanitation in connection with gastrointestinal disease.	
Knowledge about prevention of leading causes of death: cardiac disease, circulatory diseases, cancer	Do you watch your fat intake when you cook or eat out? Do you realize what high fats and cholesterol in your blood do to your blood vessels? How does exercise increase your blood circulation to your heart muscle? How are the effects of stress and smoking on your blood vessels similar?	• List measures of diet and exercise related to cardiac and circulatory disease prevention. • Explain the relationship of smoking to cardiac and circulatory disease and cancer. • Outline the effect of coffee on the body. • Explain the relationship of stress to above diseases. • Plan for regular Pap smear	Diet and exercise related to cardiac and circulatory disease prevention. Effects of smoking and coffee drinking. Effects of stress. Effects of environmental pollution as far as recognized. Value of Pap smear for prevention of cervical cancer.
Knowledge about prevention of other chronic conditions: lung disease, chronic alcohol abuse, obesity	How does smoking affect your lung tissue? Do you know any chronic alcoholics? What are they like? Have they changed physically over time? What is the reason why dieting does not work in many cases of obesity?	• Explain the effect of smoking and air pollution on lung disease. • Explain effects of alcohol on liver, intestines, brain, heart, and so on. • Outline relationship between circulation, heart activity, and body weight. • Describe symptoms and progression of these conditions.	Nature, etiology, and outcome of chronic condition mentioned. Effect of alcohol, smoking, and excessive eating. Community resources related to chronic condition Emotional factors involved.

REFERENCES

Aguilera DC, Messick JM: *Crisis Intervention: Theory and Methodology.* St Louis, Mosby, 1974.

Haber J, Leach AM, Schudy SM, Flynn BS: *Comprehensive Psychiatric Nursing.* New York, McGraw-Hill, 1978.

Holmes TH, Rahe RH: The social readjustment rating scale, *Journal of Psychosomatic Research,* 2: 213, 1967.

Levi L: *Stress and Distress in Response to Psychosocial Stimuli.* New York, Pergamon Press, 1972.

Pasquali EA, Alesi EG, Arnold HM, DeBasio N: *Mental Health Nursing: A Bio-Psycho-Cultural Approach.* St Louis, Mosby, 1981.

Selye H: *The Stress of Life.* New York, McGraw-Hill, 1956.

Wolff H: *Stress and Disease.* Springfield, Ill, Charles C Thomas, 1953.

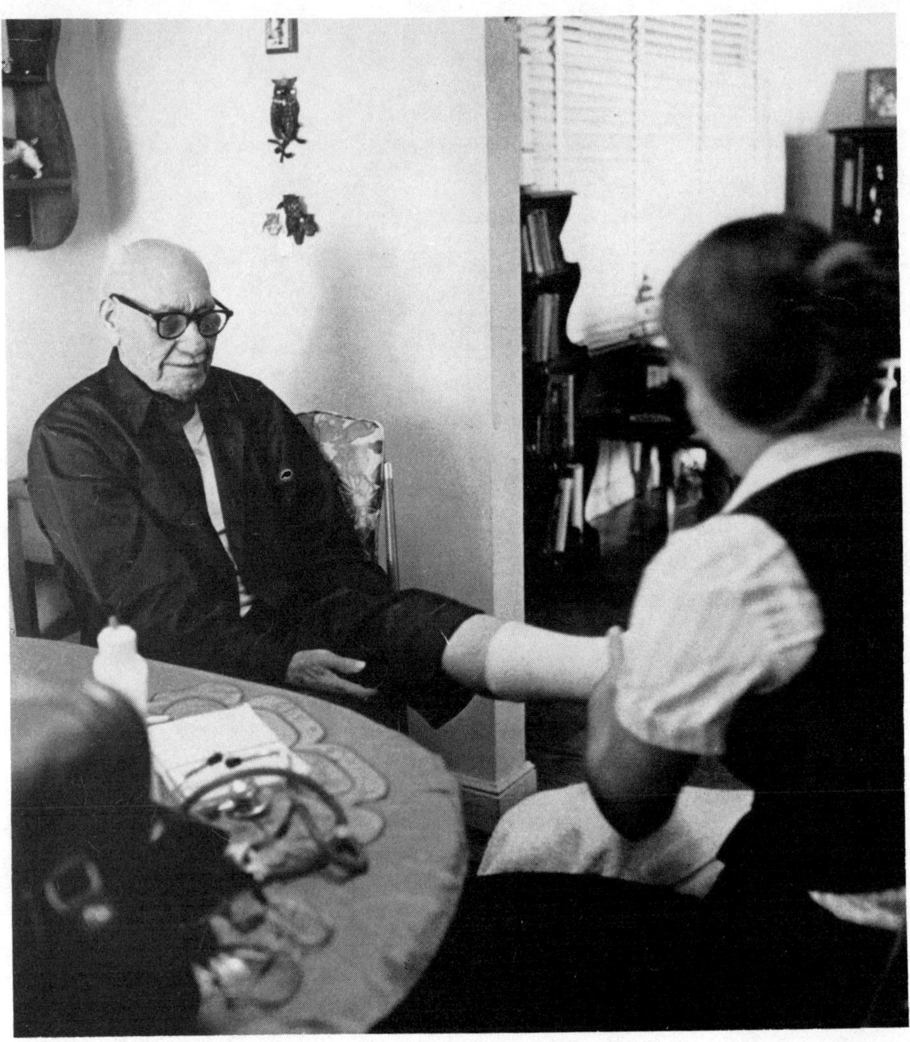

GEORGE FRYE

5

Secondary Prevention: Teaching Families with Illnesses

Primary prevention teaching serves the needs of the healthy family and helps increase their awareness about lifestyle, health, and illness prevention. Secondary prevention, however, is geared to families that have members with physical or emotional problems.

Secondary prevention teaching is practically inseparable from the implementation of the care plan, as described in Chapters 1 and 2. In the Fox family's case, it involves all the teaching needed for family and friends to understand Robert's diabetes and maintenance regime, Mrs. Fox's high blood pressure, and Robert's brother's alcohol abuse. Substance abuse teaching is much like the process mentioned under primary care teaching, but its focus is somewhat different: instead of talking about the harmful effects of other drugs on the body in order to discourage people from consuming them, the nurse describes the drug abuser's symptoms, the physiological changes that have led to them, and the prognosis if no change occurs. Thus, secondary prevention teaching centers around the person affected by the disease, and the person and family are involved in describing symptoms, asking questions, and giving feedback. Sometimes, the nurse may use pictures or plastic models to compare affected organs with healthy ones, in order to break down the denial of a person who seems unwilling to listen; this technique works best if done in the presence of the family, and true concern and empathy is expressed by the family members.

As mentioned previously, secondary prevention teaching involves teaching coupled with the performance of nursing care procedures. For many families of patients discharged from the hospital, the community health nurse may find that teaching of care-taking procedures deserves first priority. The nurse may have to explain such methods as wound irrigations, decubitus care, or other procedures that we cannot go into here but that are available in a fundamental nursing book. Although principles of sterility have to be maintained, because the equipment is often less sophisticated than that used in the hospital, the nurse and family may need to exercise ingenuity in using whatever equipment and supplies are available—pots and pans, spoons, towels, pillows, and so on—or finding them through community resources.

The nurse must teach not only procedures but also principles, so that the family understands why things must be done a certain way. In addition, the expected outcome of the procedure must be explained, and the family should know the reason for doing the procedure, the physiological processes involved, and how the procedure influences such processes. Thus, the nurse must teach about the disease in general, how it affects the client's body and mind, what the prognosis is, and what can be done by client and family to prevent permanent damage. The teaching content should thus include all areas listed in Table 5-1.

THE INITIAL VISIT: EXPLAINING DISEASE-RELATED PROCEDURES

When visiting for the first time a family with a member in need of physical care, the nurse's first concern, obviously, is to make sure that the ill person receives adequate care, and the preliminary assessment should therefore focus only on this. If the client has been discharged from a progressive teaching hospital, the family may already have been instructed in patient care; indeed, the members may have been involved in caring for the ill person in the hospital. However, even for a well-instructed family, the first day at home presents a shock. The equipment is no longer readily available, and there is no nurse to be called if the ill person is uncomfortable. Consequently, the community health nurse is usually received in the home with feelings of relief.

At that time it is important that the nurse provide an atmosphere of calmness and confidence, listen to any outpourings of anxiety and problems encountered since the hospital discharge, and provide whatever is needed to make the patient comfortable. Then the necessary assessment can be made.

First, the nurse should look at the doctor's orders and the equipment on hand, inventory supplies to be sure they are sufficient for the next few

TABLE 5-1. OVERVIEW OF SECONDARY PREVENTION TEACHING AREAS

1. Method of nursing care procedures
   a. Equipment needed
      - household equipment
      - special equipment, where to buy cheapest, where to rent, what agencies lend out free
      - bandages, and so on, disposable or reusable, what and where to purchase
      Consider insurance coverage and financial situation in making decisions about purchase of sophisticated equipment
   b. Use of equipment
      - step-by-step instruction in how to do procedure
      - principles involved in procedure
   c. Aim of procedure
      - expected result, immediately and over time
      - physiological processes involved
      - pain involved
      - projected time involved until discontinuation of procedure
2. Procedures for meeting physical needs and comfort
   Repeat above steps
3. Disease process in general
   - expected symptoms
   - physiological processes involved
   - pain involved
   - outcome, prognosis
   - effect on emotional well-being
   - expected permanent physical damage
   - avoidable permanent damage and ways to prevent it
   - effects on family members

---

days, and collect necessary household equipment such as scissors and towels. Next the nurse should assess who has responsibility for care, giving the patient as much of it as possible. If the client is not emotionally ready to look at wounds or handle care procedures, he or she should be helped to do so.

Instruction in Procedure

While equipment is being boiled for sterilization, the nurse should discuss the procedure with the patient and the person in charge. The assessment should take into account who has previously been doing the procedure and how efficiently, and what aspects are different between the hospital environment and home. By basing his or her teaching on the assessment, the nurse is better able to show how the procedure can be made easier (for example, by arranging furniture or raising the foot end of the mattress with cushions) and how the environment can be protected (such as by covering the bed with a plastic table cloth).

The procedure itself should be discussed, with the family person in charge describing it step by step and the nurse asking questions to make sure the principles are understood. This is especially important if sterile procedure is involved. The care giver needs to know about the sterile field, sources of contamination, which objects need to be sterile, and at what point they are considered clean.

After the instruments and dressings are sterile and ready, the nurse may demonstrate the procedure or let the family member proceed with it, depending on the level of confidence exhibited during the previous discussion. Either way, while the dressing change is performed, the nurse announces step by step what needs to be done, how it needs to be done, and why it needs to be done that way. A certain flexibility should be allowed, with the care giver being allowed to try better ways of working as long as they are based on the scientific principles involved, which need to be stressed to both the person in charge as well as the patient. Patients should be informed even if they take no part in the actual treatment procedure; by knowing what needs to be done, they stay in control over what is happening to their bodies and can advise the care giver on ways to proceed with least discomfort.

Determining Physical Needs

After the procedure is completed, the patient's physical needs should be discussed in detail: How does the family and the patient take care of his or her need for food, drink, elimination, exercise, positioning, cleanliness, dental care, skin care, hair care, and so on? Although emotional needs and safety needs are equally important, the ill person's physical needs are of greatest priority and need to be discussed during the first visit. Other needs may wait until the next visit, if the home is a reasonably safe place.

In complex cases, the family needs to be helped to find equipment such as hospital bed, wheelchair, and the like. Usually, however, the tasks of transferring a person from bed to chair, rolling him or her over in bed, giving regular massages and skin care are taught without difficulty. All activities of daily living need to be looked at during the first visit, and the nurse should continuously assess whether the client is understanding instructions by letting him or her repeat back what has been taught and by letting the care giver actually practice what was taught.

As described in Chapter 1, other physical needs such as diet, fluid intake, and rest and activity are covered in a general assessment, during a subsequent visit. However, the factors listed in Table 1-8 are of utmost importance and should be considered in the first visit in order to ensure adequate care for the ill family member.

The teaching plan will determine how much time and effort should be devoted to instructing the care giver. The nurse should assess the care giver's background in patient care and previous experience in order to avoid unnecessary teaching of techniques and to determine whether the care giver's intelligence level, memory, and understanding of the ill person's condition are adequate to the task. If families have minimal reading skills, they may have difficulty understanding instructions on use of equipment; the nurse may be obliged to make sketches for them and to drill them so they memorize the procedure. If families have too many child care or work obligations, they may need help dividing up responsibilities among different family members or scheduling treatments around other routines of the day. They may also need other assistance such as home-health aides to do a bath in the morning or volunteers to go shopping.

Summary of First Visit

In summary, the nurse's first visit to a family with an ill or recuperating member is usually an extensive one. The purpose is to start the family out on an adequate care-giving routine, to ensure there are adequate materials and equipment, and to teach the necessary procedures. The nurse also teaches the ability, motivation, and emotional factors related to the care of the ill person and the responsibility as well as the changes in roles and division of labor within the family. The nurse should terminate the visit satisfied that the family is confident enough to carry on independently until the next planned visit, has demonstrated the skills involved in the procedures, has verbally expressed understanding of the underlying principles, and has shown genuine concern for the client and willingness to help. Any sign of confusion, extreme nervousness, or inability to remember may indicate that the family's resources for coping are overtaxed and that further help is needed, such as the support of a member of the extended family, a friend, or a neighbor. Often giving permission to call the nursing service during the night or an emergency medical service provides sufficient reassurance.

The initial assessment areas directly related to the disease process and care of the ill member are outlined in Tables 1-7 and 1-8 as well as in Table 5-1. Tables 5-2 through 5-4 attempt to clarify assessment and teach-

TABLE 5-2. DISEASE-RELATED CARE PROCEDURES

ASSESSMENT AREAS	SAMPLE QUESTIONS	CLIENT OBJECTIVES	TEACHING AREAS
		At the end of the teaching sessions the family will:	
Knowledge of purpose of treatment	Did the doctor tell you what this procedure is good for? Does this procedure help your body to get better?	• Understand the purpose of prescribed procedures. • Explain the physiological processes demanding the procedures. • Outline the effects of the procedures on the body.	Nature of procedure. Purpose of procedure. Procedure in relation to disease processes.
Availability and condition of equipment needed Ability of care giver to purchase, maintain, and ready equipment for the procedure	Do you have a pot to sterilize these instruments or big enough to keep them covered with water? What do you have in the house that we could use to protect the bed? Do you have a plastic cloth?	• Have suitable equipment ready for procedure. • Purchase equipment needed and replenish used materials. • Maintain equipment in working order.	Suitability of household equipment. Special equipment, what and how much needed. Where to purchase or rent. Maintenance of equipment and preparation for procedure.
Knowledge and skills relative to maintenance and preparation of equipment	Do you know the purpose of boiling the instruments? What do you do next when the instruments are sterile? Where do you keep the instruments between dressing changes?	• Efficiently prepare equipment for the procedure.	Principles involved in maintenance and preparation of equipment for procedure.
Knowledge and skills relative to use of the equip-	How did you do this in the hospital?	• Diligently perform procedure. • Explain why procedure is done a certain way.	Step-by-step instruction of procedure.

ment and performing the procedure What is the safest way to use these assets?			Principles involved. Errors to be avoided.
Possibility of ill person's involvement	Have you done any part of this procedure yourself when you were in the hospital? How do you feel about looking at your wound? If you are positioned right, would you be able to reach down to your leg to remove the dressing?	• Involve the ill family member as much as his condition permits.	Measures to ease self-care: positioning, arrangement of supplies and equipment.
Knowledge of expected outcome related to procedure	Do you know how this procedure works to get you better?	• State what outcome is expected owing to procedure.	Expected outcome related to procedure.
Knowledge of physiological processes related to procedure	What do you expect to happen as a result of this treatment?	• Explain how procedure affects physiological processes.	Physiological changes induced by disease and procedure.
Knowledge of pain involved	Have you ever had a similar treatment? Did it hurt?	• State awareness of pain relative to procedure.	Pain to be expected due to procedure.
Client's knowledge of projected time until discontinuation of procedure	How long do you think this treatment needs to be continued?	• State approximately how long the treatment needs to be continued.	Time schedule, if possible to assess.

TABLE 5-3. COMFORT MEASURES

ASSESSMENT AREAS	SAMPLE QUESTIONS	CLIENT OBJECTIVES	TEACHING AREAS
		At the end of the teaching sessions the family will:	
Knowledge of family regarding position Skill of family in positioning Equipment available for positioning	What is the most comfortable position for his hand? Where do you place this pillow when you turn him over? Why would you want the pillow under his shoulders as well as under the head? Would you have a big box we could cut out and put over his feet to take the weight of the sheets off them?	• Explain the principles of positioning. • Will be skilled in positioning the ill member. • Have necessary equipment for effective positioning.	Bedridden client: • Turning techniques • Positioning on back, sides, possibly on abdomen Partially ambulatory client: • Same as above • Transfer into chair or wheelchair Positioning in sitting position.
Family's awareness of cleanliness Ability to change bed and patient's clothes Ability to give bath, dental care, skin care, hair care	Are you comfortable giving him a bath or do you need help? How did you manage to change the sheets last night? Were you able to remove his dental plates?	• State role of cleanliness and hygiene in the healing process. • Keep patient, his bed and his surroundings clean. • Give satisfactory skin, dental and hair care.	Hygiene: • Partial or complete sponge bath • Methods of changing sheets with patient in bed • Skin, dental, hair care
Possibility of ill person's involvement	See Table 5-2.		
Purchase and maintenance of equipment	See Table 5-2.		

TABLE 5-4. CARE PROCEDURES RELATED TO ELIMINATION

ASSESSMENT AREAS	SAMPLE QUESTIONS	CLIENT OBJECTIVES	TEACHING AREAS
Familiarity of family with bedpan procedure (enemas, colostomy care, and so on; see Table 5-1) Comfort of patient regarding elimination Ability to transfer to toilet seat Awareness of patient's regular elimination patterns Knowledge of measures to prevent constipation, gas, or diarrhea		*At the end of the teaching sessions the family will:* • Be skilled in handling bedpan and urinal, causing minimal discomfort to patient. • Be able to transfer the partially ambulatory patient to toilet seat comfortably. • Provide as much privacy and comfort as possible for elimination. • Keep track of elimination pattern and notice irregularities. • Use measures to prevent constipation such as fluids and diet, exercise, suppositories, if indicated.	Handling bedpans and urinals and keeping them clean. Positioning patient on the bedpan. Provide privacy. Transferring to toilet seat. Usual elimination patterns. Keeping record. Diet with regard to elimination. Fluids with regard to elimination. Use of laxatives if indicated.
Purchase and maintenance of equipment	See Table 5-2.		

ing needs in the area of nursing care procedures explained previously. The teaching plan concentrates on the disease process and its effect on patient and family.

SUBSEQUENT VISITS

The next few visits should be used to reinforce the teaching done during the first visit. The family should be checked that the prescribed procedures are being performed with diligence and understanding. The purpose of the procedures, their rationale, and the body's physiological response should be taught over one or more sessions. The family needs to be told about how long the procedures should be performed and how painful they are for the patient, who should be included in any discussion about pain since he or she can best state what it feels like and what might lessen it.

Both family and patient also need to be told more about the disease process itself. The nurse should ask what the family was told by doctors or nurses in the hospital and allow them to ask questions. Although the nurse may be unfamiliar with the problem or not have enough detail in the record to be able to answer (and certainly should not for ethical and legal reasons, if not enough information is available), he or she should promise to bring the answer on the next visit. In order to gain the family's trust, the nurse needs to follow through with this promise under all circumstances, and so should make it a point to jot down such questions in a notebook. If the physician has not fully instructed the client about the nature of his or her condition, the nurse should ask the client to discuss the matter further with the doctor. If the doctor is evasive in the first place, the nurse should try to discuss it with the doctor, and ask him or her to inform the client. The nurse can then, at least, let the client know of his or her efforts.

To teach the disease process, the nurse should use printed material, such as booklets and pamphlets, or photocopy relevant pages from medical or nursing books. To avoid later incidents of a doctor or family member who was absent during the session blaming the nurse for giving out false information, the nurse should list all printed material used in the client record and insert copies of self-made tables, diagrams, and instruction sheets into the record. If the teaching material brought by the nurse differs from the information received from the doctor, as recalled by the family, the nurse should hold off teaching that particular area until the discrepancy is clarified by the doctor. This protects not only the nurse but also the client and family, who may be confused about different kinds of information received from various health professionals, friends with the same problem, or other well-meaning individuals. Especially if the teaching involves undoing misconceptions, cultural beliefs, and superstitions, the nurse gains most credibility by presenting material supported by pamphlets, books, posters, and other audiovisual material. Chapter 9 will elaborate on teaching techniques more fully.

Every ill person wants to know what symptoms are expected in the course of the disease, the pain involved, and the outcome or prognosis. Since the answers depend on many individual variables, it is advisable in most cases for the nurse specifically to ask the doctor at the time of the referral. If the questions can be answered with any certainty, the nurse should have the answers ready on the first visit to the family, since these questions will be asked by the family eventually and since the nurse needs to gain the family's trust in order to ensure their cooperation and participation in the teaching process. The family will certainly be more impressed by a nurse who states she has talked to Dr. X and understands the following facts about the disease than by one who says, "Why don't you ask the doctor on your next visit?"

After the prognosis has been discussed and the family and patient are knowledgeable about the direction in which they are going, the nurse needs to outline measures that should be taken to speed recovery, minimize permanent damage, and increase the patient's comfort. Such measures should be presented in a positive way. As we will discuss in Chapter 9, learning and compliance will be better if the nurse uses positive reinforcement of the family's attempts to help the patient and then adds suggestions as to how it could be done even better. Threatening the family with the consequences that might happen if they do not comply easily destroys a trust relationship.

One aspect of the disease process that is often grossly neglected by health care professionals is the emotional responses of a patient to be expected after a physical trauma. Although the mechanism of such reactions is not entirely understood, research suggests that damage to body tissue causes changes within the stress response system, the endocrine mechanism located in the central nervous system (Selye, 1956). Clients undergoing surgery or recuperating from a serious illness, therefore, often react emotionally to the physical trauma, but often such a reaction takes the family by surprise, and neither the patient nor the family can explain what is going on. For example, in spite of a good prognosis and rapid progress, a recuperating person may be depressed a few days after hospital discharge or turn irritable and moody and get angry at the family for not being more helpful or for bothering him all the time. After a short time the family may feel resentful and hurt, and the recuperating family member may suspect that something is seriously wrong or is disturbed about not being able to control his or her emotions.

It is not known why certain people have more severe symptoms while others just feel tired and rest more. People who seem to be more vulnerable are the ones who get better fast, are discharged from the hospital early, and overtax their physical ability by staying up too long and by undertaking too many activities too soon after the illness. The depressive reaction may shock everyone, but it is actually a defense of the "mistreated" body, which needs time and rest to replenish resources.

Such emotional response may lead to family friction and possibly lasting damage in family relationships, especially if the family interaction and communication patterns were less than ideal to begin with. A great deal can be done to prevent this, however. The possibility of such a reaction should be anticipated in all postoperative, postpartum, and posthospitalization teaching. The nurse needs to assess carefully the activity level and rest pattern of the recuperating client. Teaching relaxation techniques and regular nap times and working out ways to reduce responsibilities with household work or children should take high priority in the hard-striving, "Type A" individual described in the stress literature (Friedman, 1969; Friedman and Rosenbaum, 1974).

Often the most devastating results happen simply because of ignorance and resulting worries that something is seriously wrong, as well as guilt feelings about impulsive and abusive behavior. The nurse's simple assurance that a depressive reaction is normal may actually restore harmony in a family that accepts such behavior and blames no one. Patients need to hear they are normal persons; giving this assurance should always be the nurse's first step of intervention.

The last aspect with regard to the teaching process concerns the involvement of care. Because the family needs to be able to clearly understand what is asked from them, the nurse should discuss with them their commitment and motivation in the context of reality. Problems should be looked at both in their present and future perspectives. The question as to how much stress a family member can tolerate without overload may be hard to answer, but certainly enough help secured initially will avoid burnout, as will finding other outlets for the care providers to help them meet their own needs. To plan efficient care, each family member needs to be assessed individually.

Subsequent visits should be used to do an extended assessment, as described in Chapter 1. All areas need to be covered, and the patient as well as all other family members should be included in the assessment.

In contrast to the assessment done for the purpose of primary prevention, the areas should be looked at from two perspectives—the state of the area before illness occurred, and the present state. One more perspective also must be added, the optimal state. The aim of teaching is to return the client as much as possible to the initial level of functioning, provided that state was satisfactory before the illness. If it was not satisfactory, teaching needs eventually to go beyond that level, to the optimal state. Unless the initial level of functioning is defined, however, nursing objectives for the optimal state will be hard to construct. The initial level of functioning is assessed in order to understand the client's potential as well as actual teaching needs.

The problems or nursing diagnoses are defined in terms of discrepancy between the optimal and the present level of functioning. The assessed discrepancies in turn need to be categorized into either fixed or avoidable problems, and the teaching plan should attempt to find measures to modify the impact of the fixed problems and find treatments and solutions for the avoidable problems.

THE SECONDARY PREVENTION PROCESS

The following example may help clarify the planning of the teaching process. The principal points are summarized in Table 5-5.

The patient is being treated for high blood pressure, which was discovered when she was hospitalized for a left radical mastectomy. Although she has recovered well, the change in her diet habits probably reflects the combined effect of preventive radiation treatment and postsurgical depression, anxiety, and insecurity. She does not feel hungry and is frequently nauseated; however, eating dry bread seems to have a soothing effect on her stomach, and so she eats a piece of bread as frequently as every half hour, though neglecting regular balanced meals. She seems to deny the importance of controlling her hypertension and will eat high-sodium foods such as canned spaghetti instead of making a conscious effort at meal planning.

In setting up objectives, the nurse needs to look at change necessitated by the fixed problem (hypertension) and temporary problems (radiation effects). The prior level of functioning needs to be taken into consideration. Previous eating habits were better than the present ones, but they were not ideal, and the hypertension means they need to be stricter. The client needs to follow a diet for salt control and weight control; however, her temporary problem of radiation sickness and her emotional problems have intervened and made it impossible to follow through with the diet.

TABLE 5-5. DIET AND FLUIDS

ASSESSMENT DATA PRIOR TO ILLNESS	PRESENT TIME	CLIENT OBJECTIVES	TEACHING AREAS
		At the end of the teaching sessions the client will:	
Some basic knowledge of food groups Consciously included a vegetable or fruit in every meal Ate reasonable quantities of food except for 3–4 slices of bread or large amounts of macaroni with meals Overweight 20 lb	Sporadically eats canned goods and frozen vegetables. Not always balanced. Quantities hard to determine. Eats little at a time but often. Frequently eats a piece of bread but has no urge to add anything else. No weight loss. Prescribed 1500 calorie no added salt diet. Lacks knowledge of foods with high salt content.	• Demonstrate good working knowledge of the four food groups. • Adhere to regular meal times. • Plan meals. • Understand and use exchange lists. • Include foods from every food group. • Recognize and avoid foods high in salt.	The basic fours. Foods high in salt. Meal planning with exchange lists for calorie control. Use previous meal pattern composition of meals. Carbohydrates. Weight control.
Drank 8–10 cups of coffee per day One glass of water with meals Small glass of milk before bed No alcoholic beverages	Still drinks same amount of coffee; states that she needs it to get going. Occasional glass of water. No more milk; no longer tastes good. Doctor did not put restriction on coffee.	• Reduce the coffee intake to 2–3 cups per day (goal set by client). • Increase water intake moderately. • Substitute milk with other dairy products.	Effect of coffee on blood vessels and heart. Regular fluid needs of body. Fluids and hypertension. Substitutes for milk.

Snacking moderate: occasional cookie and popcorn in evenings Regular three meals	No regular pattern. Meals skipped. Snacking provides main nutrition.	• Limit snacking on bread. • Substitute bread with other nutritious foods and change in eating schedule. • Plan 6 small meals per day, balanced diet—as long as on radiation treatment.	Spacing of meals. Effect of radiation on GI system. Balancing of 6 small meals.
Liked most foods Disliked some vegetables: broccoli, brussel sprouts and cabbage Liked sweets Liked milk and milk products Special liking for starch foods	Has difficulties with meats especially if they need to be chewed. Eats hamburger meat and hot dogs, chicken, and fish. Fruits and vegetables no change. Sweets lost attraction. Starch foods most liked and eaten almost exclusively. Lost taste for milk. Still eats cheese.	• Integrate liked foods from all food groups into planned meals.	Help in integrating likes into meal plan.
Used to eat in kitchen only. Enjoyed food. Ate slowly. Ate with company 3 times per week	Does not sit down to eat bread. If meal is fixed she eats in the kitchen. Eats very slowly, observing how stomach reacts to food. No more company; afraid she might vomit.	• Feel less anxious about eating. • Be comfortable eating with friends. • Eat 6 meals in the kitchen.	Explore anxiety about food. Relate fears to self-image.
Enjoyed food. Food had traditional and cultural meaning	Frustrated. No longer likes food or self.	• Accept present problem as temporary. • Express the meaning of food. • Try out different kinds of food in small amounts. • Have a satisfactory body image.	Help express problem.

This means the nurse should explore other areas and help the client resolve her emotional problems, in order to gain her compliance.

The client is in need of diet teaching, meal planning, and the elimination of salty foods, but she will not be receptive to this teaching until her other needs are met as well and she is no longer plagued by excessive anxiety about possible cancer. If the nurse has been able to gain her confidence by presenting facts and prognosis about her disease and by being an empathetic listener, the client may be ready for teaching in the diet area. Nurse and client first need to agree on a set of objectives. The nurse then should look at the client's prior level of functioning in the dietary area. The nurse can point out to the client what diet aspects she has handled well in the past and let her explain how she did the diet planning before her illness. Together they should look at the dynamics and explore which diet practice could be transferred to the present. If, for example, the client has used a menu book in the past, could it also be used now? If she frequently had invited guests over in order to make cooking more attractive, what keeps her from doing it now?

Because she had been eating three meals a day, it seems likely that she eventually will resume her old routine. To get around the problem of nausea, the client agrees to a compromise of six meals that include not only bread but also foods from the meat, milk, or fruit and vegetable groups. Her likes and dislikes are incorporated in suggestions for the preparation of these meals. The choice of foods also depends on the client's routine, time available, and her willingness to prepare meals. These factors are assessed in the "activity and rest patterns" area and are carried over to diet teaching. If the client does not get up until noon, the nurse may propose a light lunch for a starter and a late-night meal before going to bed. If the client is actively doing volunteer work for the community in the afternoons, she cannot cook her midafternoon meal, but she may be willing to take some cottage cheese and an apple along. In short, diet suggestions are worthless unless they are discussed in the context of the client's routine and motivation to prepare foods. The success rate is likely to be greater if the client actively participates in the problem-solving process by suggesting the foods she might like and might be able to prepare.

The assessment and teaching for all other assessment areas should be done in similar fashion. While going through the problem-solving process and finding ways to meet the ill client's needs together with patient and family, the nurse will see that the client's needs cannot be fully met unless the whole family can adjust successfully to the new tasks and routine and meet their own needs. The individual assessment of the family members involved in care and the family assessment both provide the nurse with valuable information. If in both assessments data is available describing conditions prior to the illness and at present, the nurse will have a fairly clear picture of the extent of adjustment the family needs to make.

The assessments will also tell how far the adjustment has proceeded up to the present point and where the difficulties lie. For example, if a wife caring for her sick husband has previously held a job with a considerable amount of responsibility and contact with different people, she may experience depression and irritability and be angry at doctors or nurses for not responding quickly enough to her demands. Yet such a change may cause her some guilt, since her values may tell her that she should be a dedicated wife bearing her burden with dignity and not let her husband feel any of her stress. A nurse may be alerted to the problem not only by the wife's anger and demands but also by the discrepancy between her previous and present lifestyles and will realize she is probably not fulfilling her needs for self-esteem and esteem by others by caring for her husband, especially if she feels her care is incompetent and her security is threatened by her husband's uncertain prognosis.

To be helpful to the family, the nurse needs to go through the process of data integration described in Chapter 2 and understand how the changes brought about by the husband's illness influence the system and within it the well-being of all family members. A comprehensive care plan, therefore, not only provides good physical care and emotional support for the ill member but helps other family members to find as much fulfillment and self-esteem as possible within their new life. The care plan also provides for relief for family members to meet needs that are impossible to fulfill within the care-giving role, especially if the situation involves high tension. The nurse needs to mobilize diverse resources to help the family—financial, emotional, spiritual, and physical help with care. Often this kind of teaching involves informing the family about the nature of their stress, of letting them know that emotional reactions to stress are normal and expected. Care providers also need to be told they still have the right to lead their own lives, that they need not sacrifice all personal satisfaction for the sake of the ill member.

The Kent Family Example

Culture and values strongly influence attitudes of the family and often create overwhelming conflicts within it, which destroy the family harmony and affect the care of the ill member. Such an example is the Kent family. Son Bobby, age 9, has cystic fibrosis; the second son, Scott, age 5, is healthy. Mrs. Kent has given excellent care to Bobby ever since his condition was diagnosed at age 5 months. Previously Mrs. Kent had been a school teacher and had enjoyed her profession very much. However, she never went back to work after Bobby's birth, because she felt an obligation to dedicate her life to him—in part because she felt guilty about being the cause of Bobby's disease. A strong, independent woman, Mrs. Kent handles crises extremely well and feels she does not need help from others. Her mother told her in early childhood that a woman's burden was heavy, but that women were made to bear it and were not to complain. Her mother had religion to comfort her and give her strength; Mrs. Kent, on the other hand, feels alienated from the church and has rejected any kind of religious involvement.

The family functioned reasonably well in the past, but at present problems appear to be getting worse, and Mrs. Kent is running out of energy and resources. Moody and depressed, she often retreats to her bedroom to cry. When she is feeling self-pity, she goes through a process of comparing herself to all of her friends and acquaintances who have been successful with careers, are involved in community activities, or are engaged in many leisure activities, travel, and social engagements. Mrs. Kent feels isolated; her life is Bobby. She cannot relate well to her friends, since she feels she is different and they will not understand her depression. She does not tell them either, since the only thing that keeps her going is the admiration she is getting from her friends for doing what she is doing. How could she admit that she is not doing as well as she should? Mrs. Kent is torn between resentment about not being a liberated woman, not living to her full potential, not getting fun out of life, and her values dictating her to "do her duty."

Mr. Kent feels the conflict of his wife more and more and retreats to his office, working overtime or on weekends. Often he feels like a stranger in the house, and when he pursues his own interests because he no longer feels part of the family routine, his wife starts an argument and blames him for not caring. Scott is jealous of Bobby, especially since he is going to kindergarten. He feels that his mother wants him out of the house. He acts up frequently; beats up on Bobby, since he is now equal in strength; and gets in trouble with his mother, driving her to desperation. He openly tells Bobby that he hates him.

Bobby has begun crying a lot, blaming the family for not liking him. At one point he asked them to send him away somewhere else; although he did not really mean it, it deeply hurt Mrs. Kent's feelings, and she sat with him for a long time trying to comfort him. Bobby is also getting to a stage of development in which he resents being "Mommy's boy." He would like to be respected by other boys in school, but this is difficult, since he is sick a lot and cannot compete with them physically. Mrs. Kent attempts to counteract his sore feelings by telling him how much she loves him. However, every time he brings up unpleasant incidents from school she feels deep sadness owing to her own guilt. Bobby feels this, and so reports the incidents less often; but he feels anger toward his mother for not letting him be like others.

Recognizing this system of variables interacting with each other is the first step for nursing intervention. The nurse should explain the network to the family so that it can participate in the search for solutions and help decide which interventions would be most effective. The nurse may be able to propose some beginning measures to give Bobby more independence and responsibility and point out the needs of Mrs. Kent so that she can allow herself more opportunity for involvement outside the family, but some problems will need other professional help. The nurse might discuss with them marriage counseling or family therapy that would also include the children. Depending on the extent of Bobby's emotional problems, he may be in need of individual or group therapy. Other options might include a support group for cystic fibrosis parents, vocational counseling for Mrs. Kent, and summer camp for Bobby. After describing the available programs to them, the nurse should let them make the decisions.

In summary, the nurse and the family together should discuss every family member's needs and jointly find ways to meet these needs better. Such family teamwork is especially important, since any change in the routine of one family member will affect all others, and adjustments need to be made in the family assessment areas of "interaction" (especially roles and division of labor) and "communication" (see Chapter 1). If, for example, Mrs. Kent decides to get involved in a college program in special education, many aspects of the family routine will need to be reorganized. Mr. Kent would have to be supportive of her plan and assist her with Bobby's preventive treatments, or a babysitter would have to be trained. Bobby would have to take the responsibility of keeping track of his treatments himself. If the family cannot afford cleaning help, these chores might become a joint venture for everyone, and Bobby, too, would have his tasks to do, such as vacuuming his own room or doing his laundry.

The willingness of every family member to do his or her fair share is imperative for success. This group process may be difficult, and talking back and forth may be required until the necessary compromises are made that leave everyone satisfied. In this process the nurse needs to be a cool, impartial leader, an important mediator who can help avoid heated arguments and hurt feelings.

TABLE 5-6. STEPS OF SECONDARY PREVENTION TEACHING

Initial Visit

1. Make preliminary assessment: procedure and equipment.
2. Make assessment of care giver's involvement, skills and motivation.
3. Instruct procedures step by step; let family members perform the task.
4. Teach some rationale for procedure.
5. Teach procedure for replenishing supplies and equipment.
6. Assess physical needs and comfort of ill client.
7. Assess equipment at hand.
8. Teach comfort measures.
9. Procure equipment necessary or instruct family.
10. Assess comfort and safety of patient and family until next visit.

Subsequent Visits

1. Check and reinforce procedure teaching.
2. Teach
   - Rationale for procedure
   - Aim of procedure—expected outcome
   - Physiological processes involved
   - Pain involved
3. Teach disease process
   - Expected symptoms
   - Physiological processes
   - Pain
   - Outcome—prognosis
   - Possible effect on emotional well-being
   - Expected physical damage
   - Ways to avoid permanent damage
   - Expected involvement of family members
4. Do extended assessment of patient (see Chapter 1); include state prior to disease, state after disease, and ideal state (objectives).
5. Do extended assessment of all other family members (see Chapter 1).
6. Do family assessment (see Chapter 1).
7. Plan the care (Chapter 2); consider state prior to illness.
8. Discuss network of influencing variables with family.
9. Set objectives together with family.
10. Teach within problem areas.

The Example of the Sanders Family

In some families, values and culture are helpful influences in the matter of taking care of ill family members. The Sanders are a Black family who moved to the area 10 years ago and have adjusted well to their new community and lifestyle, in part because of a close network of friends all supporting each other.

Recently Mr. Sanders hurt his back in an accident, which requires he wear a body brace; he has difficulty moving around and needs help with his usual daily activities. As soon as he came home from the hospital, neighbors brought food and presents and offered their services to the family. Since Mrs. Sanders worked afternoons, she prevailed on two of her best friends to watch her husband during that time and to cook dinner for him and the children. The neighbors' children join them in the Sanders's home for dinner also. Mr. Sanders enjoys the company and they all have a good time, even though there is not enough room for everybody at the table and the children have to eat sitting on the couch. If Mr. Sanders needs some rest, all the children are sent away to a neighbor's house; there is a good deal of free flow among the houses in the block and sharing of family happenings.

In planning care the nurse should make use of these resources. Teaching nursing care to several people in the neighborhood may be more time consuming and it will need more periodic checking since the chance for error or omission of the treatment is greater. However, the ill client will feel happier and more at ease within his or her own environment and may well be more cooperative than with personnel from a nursing or other community agency coming in to do treatment.

Summary of the Secondary Prevention Process

Summarizing this process of teaching secondary prevention, Table 5-6 shows the steps that should be taken by the nurse.

This should be followed by a primary prevention teaching program (see Chapter 4).

REFERENCES

Friedman M: *Pathogenesis of Coronary Artery Disease.* New York, McGraw-Hill, 1969.

Friedman M, Rosenbaum RH: *Type A Behavior and Your Heart.* New York, Knopf, 1974.

Selye H: *The Stress of Life.* New York, McGraw-Hill, 1956.

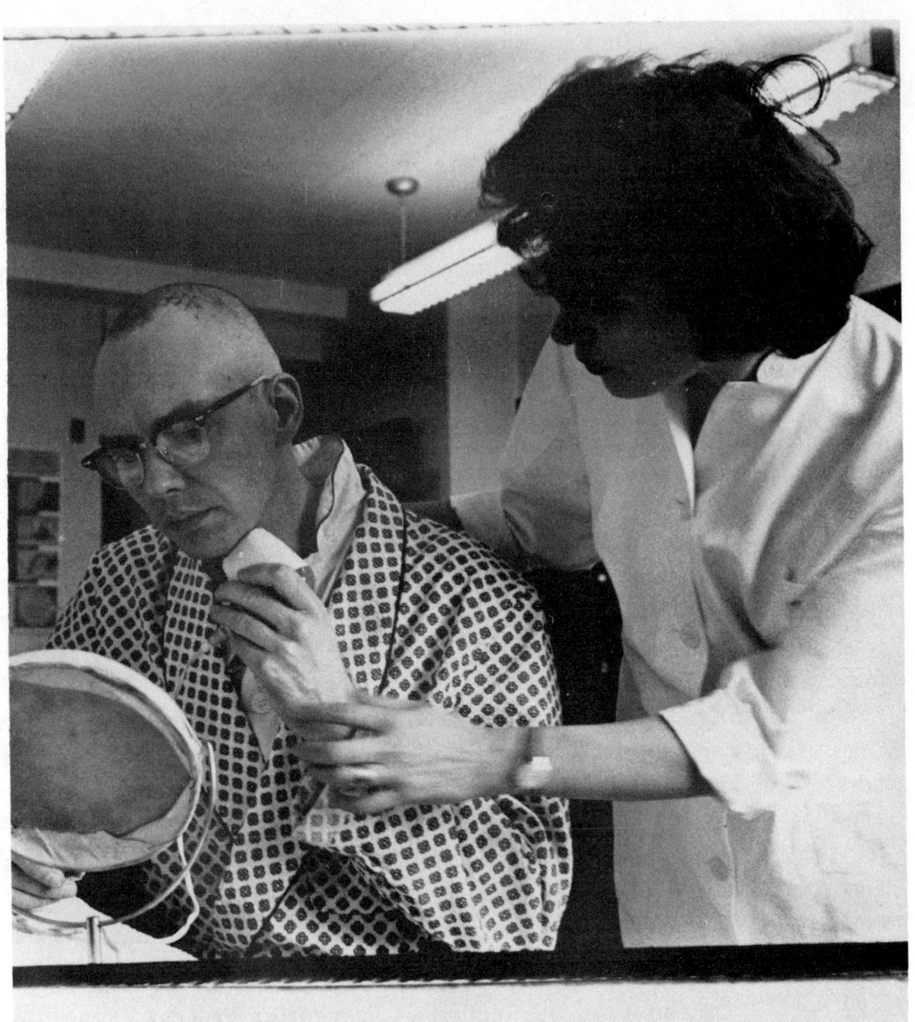

6

Tertiary Prevention: Teaching Rehabilitation

The teaching process in tertiary prevention is very similar to one in secondary prevention. The difference between the two lies in the focus of the problems. Whereas the secondary prevention teaching plan includes all areas related to the disease process, tertiary prevention encompasses the rehabilitation aspect after the illness has passed. Often tertiary prevention teaching occurs later in time, but not necessarily so. In the example of the Fox family in Chapters 1 and 2, tertiary prevention teaching was concerned with helping the family adjust to the changes that had happened in Mrs. Fox's health and pointing out ways to better use Robert's potential as well as working with Robert toward better compliance with the medical regime in order to prevent further complications.

ADDRESSING PHYSICAL AND EMOTIONAL NEEDS

The typical case a community health nurse thinks of in terms of tertiary care is the rehabilitation client, the post-CVA client, or the paraplegic. Here the rehabilitation is thought of as a regime to improve physical capabilities to reach an optimal level of independent physical functioning. The regime is usually prescribed by an orthopedist or physical therapist. The role of the community nurse in such a family is one of coordinator. Exercises need to be supervised, and cooperation has to be assured from family and patient. The family needs to be taught how to help the afflicted person with the exercises.

Many teaching needs, however, are not easily separated from secondary prevention teaching. A post-CVA client needs care such as skin care when in bed, help in transferring into a chair or toilet seat, or help with a bath, which are considered secondary prevention measures. These same measures, however, should also be taught from the perspective of tertiary prevention. Teaching the family how to give a bath should be a matter of assuring the afflicted client's maximum participation. Family members need to be made aware of the importance of brushing teeth as an exercise for hand and arm, and they should refrain from their natural urge to want to help since the process is labored and slow. For all facets of care, the client has to be carefully evaluated as to how much he or she can do for himself, or at least assist the care provider.

This leads into another aspect of tertiary care that is equally important—the emotional well-being of the client. Every experienced nurse has experienced the difference in rehabilitation results between a motivated, positively thinking client and that of a person who has given up hope. Whereas the physical part of rehabilitation may be directed by other professionals, the emotional aspect—and with it to a great extent the success of the program—rests with the client and the community health nurse. The real challenge for the nurse rests in helping the family function in harmony, making the client feel worthwhile and appreciated in spite of the handicap, and making the care givers happy with the work they are doing yet able to meet their personal needs by supporting each other and by effective communication.

PLANNING TERTIARY PREVENTION

Tertiary prevention should be kept in mind at all times with all clients recuperating from illness. When we plan secondary care by assessing the discrepancy between the previous level of functioning and the present level of functioning, we are actually thinking in terms of tertiary prevention as well. The two can hardly be separated. Primary prevention aspects may also gain importance after a bout of illness; some areas will be taught in the light of preventing the illness from recurring rather than preventing the illness altogether. An example of this is stress management. Stress management is an important area in anybody's life and is taught preventively to avoid stress-related diseases. In people who have already suffered stress-related disorders, such as a heart attack or a gastric ulcer, the same teaching gains a new focus. Since the likelihood of a recurrence of the disease is great if the factors leading to it are not modified, tertiary prevention is of major importance. This also holds true for the areas of diet and activity-rest patterns relative to stress diseases.

Because of the close relationship between secondary and tertiary prevention teaching, the planning of each follows identical steps, as described in Chapter 5, Table 5-6. If procedures are involved, the community health nurse again needs to make sure that the equipment is available and in good order and that the family knows how to use it. Teaching also involves the how-to-do of the procedures, the purpose and rationale, and comfort measures and safety precautions. Some of the procedures may pertain strictly to tertiary care, such as range-of-motion exercises or self-catheterization. Some secondary-care procedures, such as decubitus care or wound irrigation, are taught in the light of prevention of further complications as well, since they too are necessary to allow successful rehabilitation of the client.

Subsequent teaching is identical, too, but with the focus on future functioning rather than on the disease and healing processes alone. Neither in the assessment nor in the plan for teaching can the two levels of prevention be kept apart.

FAMILY DYNAMICS

The most significant difference between secondary and tertiary care lies in the family dynamics revolving around the afflicted member. In secondary prevention, the focus of care is on the disease process. The family regards the patient as passive and in need of care, and if such care is provided he or she will get better. Tertiary prevention, on the other hand, is perceived as a dynamic process spurred by the patient's own initiative to gain strength and reacquire previous skills and abilities. Whereas secondary prevention focuses on impairments, tertiary prevention builds on remaining strengths. The main object of teaching in the family area is to make the family aware of these strengths and help them reassess the process of rehabilitation on an ongoing basis. The family needs to be taught the importance of letting patients make decisions such as setting the times for their exercises, of giving patients opportunities to contribute to their care as well as to perform helpful tasks in the household if they are able to. The community health nurse should stress to the family that patient feelings of worthlessness and powerlessness lead to depression and that such depression will invariably interfere with the process of recuperation. Giving patients some autonomy, some power to make decisions, and explaining to them the necessity of their dependency in other areas may help to prevent severe depression. Communication needs to be kept open at all times. Patients need to be able to express feelings of worthlessness and they should be involved in a process of finding activities that are worthwhile and that they might like to do. Fighting such depression is relatively easy if the prognosis is favorable and the state of dependency may be regarded as transitory. Family and nurse may then stress to clients the progress they have made over time and can let them recognize that setbacks are expected and that progress needs to be looked at within a larger time frame. Such care is more easily tolerated by the family as well since they can foresee better times ahead.

SERIOUSLY ILL PATIENTS

The real challenge to the community health nurse is the family with a member who is and remains permanently disabled and dependent on others, or the member whose condition will further deteriorate and who may eventually die as a result of the affliction. Most professionals now feel that the family has the right to know the diagnosis, the expected course of the disease, and the prognosis. The doctor may want to have the sole responsibility of informing the client or may be willing to share it with the nurse. This is a touchy matter, and communication between doctor and nurse is imperative not just at the time the diagnosis is told the family, but also during the ongoing process of adaptation. Rather than expressing hostility about who has the authority to do what, the two professionals should support each other and help each other meet the family's needs. They should share important observations and alert each other to the family's strengths and problems as they appear in the course of time.

Bad news can be communicated to a family in many ways, as we will discuss in detail in Chapter 9. The nurse should keep in mind that no matter how negative the news is, there can always be something positive included about the prognosis in order to cushion the shock. A family will accept a diagnosis of terminal cancer more easily if the nurse assures them that the client's pain will be controlled carefully to provide maximum comfort and that the nurse will be assisting the family all the way through the process and help them in any way possible. A quadriplegic who has to be told that his or her paralysis will not improve owing to permanent damage to the nervous column will do better if the potential for rehabilitation is stressed rather than the disability, if the nurse tells about (or introduces) people who have successfully overcome the depression and lived to their full potential. In addition, the nurse should keep in mind that clients will accept bad news in different ways. Some will cope with denial by selectively hearing only positive information. This coping mechanism may be functional in dampening the impact of the shock, but as time passes the nurse should be aware of the need to restate the nature of the client's condition in realistic terms.

Depression will invariably set in. Often it is disguised in cheerfulness toward nurse and family but will take over during the quiet night hours or manifest itself by inability to sleep, loss of appetite, or other somatic symptoms, which at times are hard to distinguish from the symptoms of the actual disease. The nurse should expect a grief response and look for it under an elaborate system of defenses. The family too responds with grief. Changes in interaction patterns should be observed carefully and interpreted to the family in order to open up communication. Open communication is the key for the prevention of misinterpretation of behavior and resulting hard feelings. Disaster within the family can be avoided if the family members understand and expect the grief reaction, and a community nurse's empathy is often of immeasurable value.

MENTALLY ILL PATIENTS

If understanding each other's behavior is of major importance for the functioning of a family, one can easily understand why a family member with a mental health or psychiatric problem can cause turmoil and disruption within the family. With the advent of the community mental health movement in the sixties, many mental patients have been discharged back into the community and, where possible, back into their families. Today's psychiatric treatment is usually performed on an outpatient basis wherever feasible, which leaves the family with the enormous responsibility of taking care of their affected member. As a rule, the support a family gets from the community mental health agency is minimal, day treatment facilities are limited, and jobs that take into account the low tolerance for stress of the mental client are rare. A community nurse can be of great value for a family by locating the available community resources for the family or by simply listening and helping the family analyze their problem.

The Example of Donna

The example of Donna provides some insight into the many facets of daily living affected by the presence of a mental client in the family. The community health nurse gained access to Donna's family and home owing to their isolated location and their inability to pick up a new supply of medication from the community mental health agency on a regular basis. The purpose of the first visit was the delivery of these medications.

Donna and her family live in a medium size, four-bedroom home on a small lake in the country, some 20 miles from the nearest larger settlement. Donna's stepmother and father both work full time during the day. Money is no problem for the family. Their style of living is moderate but includes a few luxuries such as a motorboat, which they like to use on their lake.

Donna was admitted to the state hospital at age 15, when she was diagnosed a paranoid schizophrenic. Twenty years later, at age 35, she was discharged to her home. At the time of the visit, three years after her discharge, she was very unhappy. She complained about having to leave the state hospital. It had been her home and she had several friends whom she now misses. She does not feel welcome at home. "They are mean to me," she explains. "They don't like me." Donna spends her day in an occupational center for the handicapped assembling springs to be used in car seats. She is able to earn a few dollars a day. A bus picks her up at her house and brings her back home. Donna enjoys that part of her life. She is quite sociable and has made some friends with whom she spends coffee time and lunch break. Donna's mental condition is controlled with a maintenance dose of medication, which is monitored by the occupational center during the day and by her family on evenings and weekends.

Donna shows much anger toward her father. She demands the responsibility of taking her own pills by refusing to accept them if her father gives them to her. Her mother has been keeping entirely out of this conflict but resents having to put up with her husband's daughter. The father checks the supply of medication every evening and has realized that the morning or evening dose is skipped by Donna frequently. This has become more of a problem since Donna is afflicted with an associated seizure disorder. During the last few weeks she experienced two seizures at work. The father is angry with Donna and feels powerless. His attempts to communicate end in screaming at her for being so stubborn and irresponsible. Donna does not indicate any willingness to change.

Donna's moving back into the family has changed many facets of family life for her parents and her 15-year-old half-sister, a child of her father's present marriage who lives in the house. Even though Donna has her own room, she does not spend much time there. When home from work, she turns on the TV and stays in the family room until late at night. She chooses the TV program and the rest of the family has to watch what she watches. The family feels uncomfortable about inviting friends over since Donna will not socialize with the guests except for some one-word answers but instead continues watching TV.

On weekends Donna gets bored. There is nothing to do for her and she does not get involved in household chores. Donna likes to go to church; however, it is a half hour's drive from their home. The parents do not go. At times, one of Donna's married sisters picks her up to go to church with her. Even though Donna is told when her sister cannot make it, Donna sits by the door in her coat, and if her sister does not arrive she has a tantrum lasting some ten minutes. She then retreats into a corner of the living room where, visible to all, she stares into space for two or three hours, by which time her behavior is normalized again.

The mother tolerates her behavior without complaining openly. Spoiled as a child, even today her life has no restrictions. Her family adjusts their own life to Donna's rather than making her comply. Donna's father carries the responsibility for her. He coerces her into taking a bath and washing her hair, which seems to become a more and more tedious job. He and his other daughter take turns staying home with Donna when she decides to take a day of sick leave. This happens at least once a month owing to her severe menstrual cramps. The father is already worried about Donna's future menopause and possible changes in her behavior, and states if it gets any worse he cannot keep her home.

The reason for Donna's need to be supervised is two suicide attempts within the past three years in which she slashed her wrists. No attempts have occurred during the last six months or since Donna found the job at the occupational center.

The community nurse sees her role as a sounding board to listen to everyone's problems and eventually contribute in an effort to improve family communication and interaction patterns. After doing an assessment and going through the process of integrating the complex material into a comprehensive framework, she realizes that the coping patterns of neither Donna nor the father are in the best interests of the rest of the family. The mother's lenient attitude is perceived by Donna as a way of ignoring her. In order to feel safe, Donna needs limits set and reinforced. The father's approach is not effective either, since his controlling behavior communicates to her that he does not accept her or trust her. In his presence she does not feel like a worthy human being. Her need for autonomy and respect by others does not get satisfied either way and as a result Donna resorts to temper outbursts.

At work Donna is treated with respect. Her superior takes a few minutes each day to listen to her problems and makes certain that he comments on Donna's excellent performance. As a result, Donna accepts the limits set, such as the time limit on the coffee break or the fact that she has to take her medication. Occasionally, if she needs to be reprimanded for unacceptable behavior, Donna may resort to sulking, but no longer than 10 minutes at a time.

It seems obvious that some of these principles, if transferred to the family, would make everyone's life easier. The nurse has to use extreme caution, however. A presentation of how things *should be* handled versus how they *are* handled would most likely result in the parents being angry about being blamed for not managing Donna well and about the nurse's not understanding what their real problem is.

Based on all the factors, the nurse decides that the best way to handle the problem is by way of a family group discussion of everyone's needs and perception as to what is going on. Necessary changes will then be decided on by all family members. The involvement of the nurse is that of a group leader who will point out implications of the family situation on the proposed actions. At times, the nurse adds suggestions, after making sure they do not make the family feel it is being blamed for what is happening. The nurse's participation transmits to the family a genuine concern for their problem and understanding of everyone's position.

As a result of such nursing intervention, the family now has solved the main problems. Donna's needs are taken care of by the father's accepting her urge to regulate her regime. Positive reinforcement is used if she takes her medication and keeps herself clean. If she forgets, she is reminded by any one of the other family members in a matter-of-fact way. Donna's behavior in her free time has also improved; she had expressed the wish to invite one of her friends from work occasionally on a weekend, and this has worked wonders. Since her friend is treated well and is made to feel welcome by the family, Donna herself feels for the first time as part of the family. Since then she has made an effort to communicate with other people visiting the family and, at times, even gives them permission to turn off the TV. On one occasion Donna let her mother watch a program different from the one she had in mind, and much gratefulness was expressed by the mother. The situation is not perfect, and Donna still has her bad days; however, even those are better accepted by the family, which seems happy that Donna is actually able to observe some limits for the good of everyone.

This example shows that Donna's rehabilitation toward more effective interaction with her family has been possible with support of the nurse and mobilization of the family's own resources. The example of tertiary prevention can be applied in any family situation in which disturbances are noted, either in interaction patterns or in family communication. (Chapter 11 will have a more detailed discussion.)

CONCLUSION

In terms of the mental client, tertiary prevention involves the process of readjustment—for example, after a suicide attempt, or discharge from a mental hospital after an acute psychotic attack, or (as is the case with children) after a crisis situation is resolved and some emotional effects, usually evidenced by behavior problems, remain to be worked on. Often emotional problems resulting from another chronic condition lead to friction in the family and need to be looked at in terms of tertiary prevention as well. This is the case in conditions such as seizure disorders, hyperactivity, a physical handicap, or mental retardation.

As described in this chapter, teaching within the tertiary prevention area follows the same steps (Table 5-6) as secondary prevention teaching. However, it is focused on the dynamic process of change toward OPLOF rather than on the disease process itself. The role of the family in the teaching process is one of active participation, and the effective community health nurse is the one with skills in leading and directing the group process.

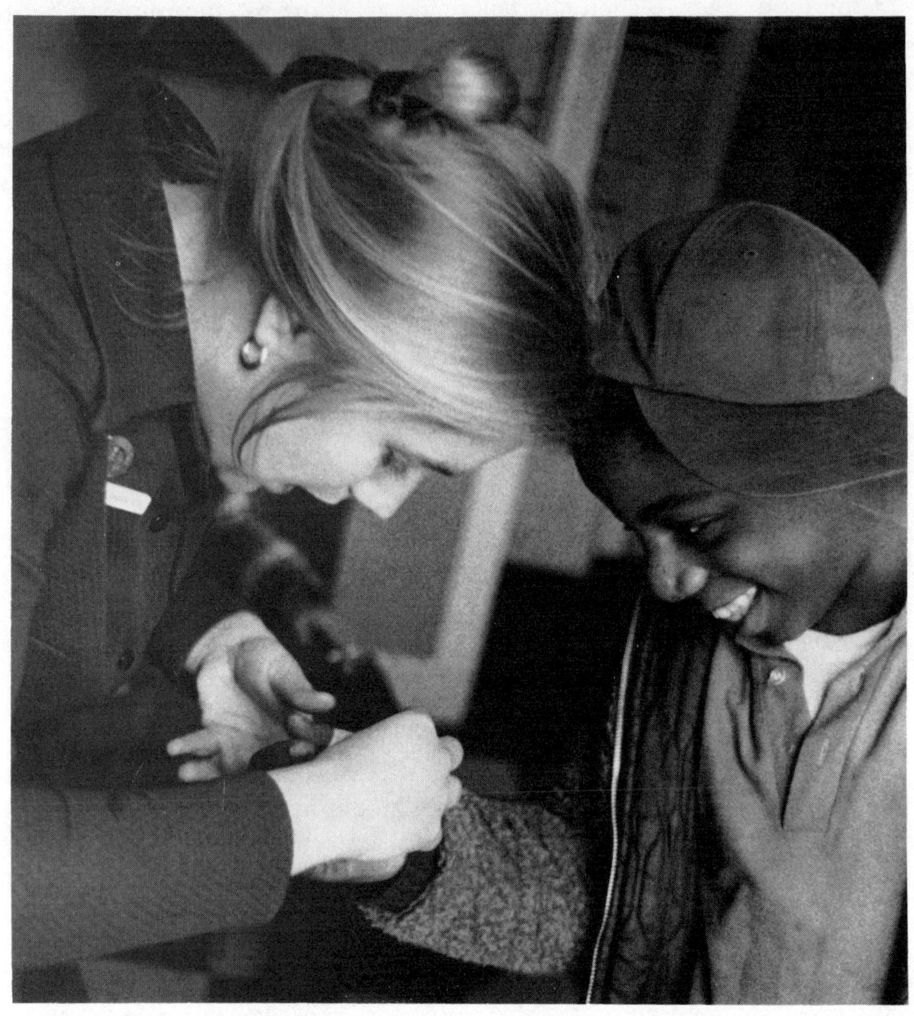

L. FLEESON/STOCK, BOSTON

III

Communication and Behavioral Dimensions of Community Nursing

EVERY ADULT & TEENAGER SHOULD BE TAUGHT TO
FIGHT V.D. WITH SOAP AND WATER
WASH
MEN: FOR BETTER PERSONAL HYGIENE WASH BEFORE SEX.
IMMEDIATELY AFTER SEX:
WOMEN:
(212) 269-5300
YOU WILL
NEVER KNOW
IF YOU'RE
CURED UNLESS
YOU RETURN
FOR YOUR
TEST
OF
CURE
KEEP ALL YOUR APPOINTMENTS
IT'S
YOUR
HEALTH
?
a woman's concern
B·D
plastic
strips
B·D
SINGLE SAMPLE
NEEDLE

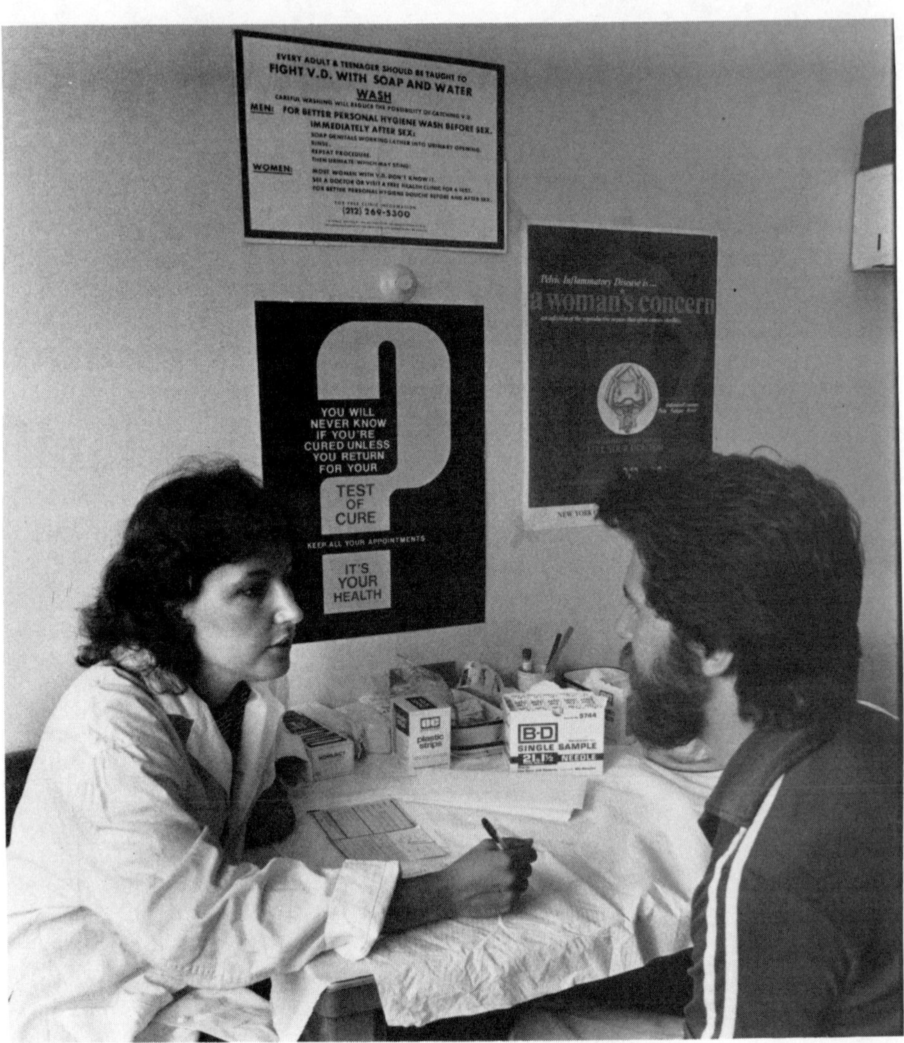

GEORGE FRYE

7

The Initial Contact

Community health nursing has been defined as a process that can occur in any community setting such as hospitals, clinics, or a client's home. In any of these settings the initial contact between client and nurse usually involves a certain amount of tension and insecurity. The tension may be minimal and may be resolved after the first word is spoken, or it may remain unchanged and even accelerate during ongoing sessions with the client. This anxiety and tension is related to several intervening factors, which will be discussed here.

In this chapter we will use the client's home setting in order to elaborate on these factors. When doing home visits, the nurse is confronted with more unknown and uncertain variables than is a nurse who functions in a familiar setting. This uncertainty is likely to produce anxiety that can only be resolved with much experience and familiarity with the community, the types of homes, and the culture of the families served. Even then, the experienced community health nurse at times encounters situations that are unexpected and require the performance of a role the nurse has not previously been practicing.

Although the chapter describes situations arising during home visits, the principles discussed can and should be applied to all community health settings, and the nurse should be consciously working on sharpening the awareness of his or her own emotional responses to the clients, the family members' looks, their behavior, and particularly their value system as expressed verbally and nonverbally.

NURSE FACTORS

At the moment of entering a client's home, the nurse experiences an emotional reaction of either immediate ease and comfort or insecurity and discomfort. The reaction is similar to what happens when a person meets someone for the first time: one experiences some like or dislike of the stranger. The brain provides instant information by using a coding system similar to the one used by a computer. The process is called *association.*

Starting at birth, everyone's brain is busy categorizing experiences in order to gain understanding of the world and its orderly processes. Theorists such as Sullivan (1953) or Berne (1961) see this process as a necessary part in gaining identity, or a *script* in Berne's terms. According to them, people learn about themselves by observing how others react to them—accept them or reject them. The young child not yet able to logically reason, since the concepts basic to the process are not learned yet, attempts to organize information about people by constructing an individual coding system. People who are friendly get coded positively and those abrupt and unfriendly get a negative evaluation. The child then finds common characteristics. If, for example, Uncle Harry, who wears a beard and glasses and has dark curly hair, is a fun person to be with, since every time he visits he brings a little surprise and lets the kids have piggyback rides, Uncle Harry's characteristics such as beard and hair get a positive mark in the coding system as well. Consequently, among a group of people, the child will unconsciously initiate interaction first with a person who has something in common with Uncle Harry or, for that matter, with any other positively coded person the child has previously encountered. Characteristics used for the coding system are manifold: hair color, shape of nose, tone of voice, smell of perfume, quality of gait, or even objects associated with the person, such as clothing, jewelry, or car.

Even in adulthood, when a stranger is met, the old coding system becomes activated. The qualities of the stranger are matched with the ones stored in the memory, and the person concludes whether the stranger should be liked or disliked. In reality, this process is not well understood since most of it happens in the subconscious mind and is much more complicated than outlined. The purpose of this schematic explanation, however, is to point out how irrational such conclusions may be. A major part of the coding system has been built up in childhood in the absence of an awareness that there is no actual relationship between the characteristics of such persons and the experiences these persons provided. Most of these associations are purely emotional and have nothing to do with rational thinking.

The reactions nurses experience when entering a client's home are similar in nature, since the brain categorizes not only people-related characteristics but also other kinds of experiences, the material environment, nature, and so on. The reaction of feeling either comfortable or ill at ease in a home is based on past experiences. The more similarity there is between a client's home and settings familiar to the nurse, the better the nurse can function. Severe contrast is shocking and creates insecurity about the role the nurse is expected to play.

Values interfere with the nurse's effectiveness as well. There is much similarity between values and the association and conclusions drawn about the nature of people and things. Values, too, are formed in a process started very early in childhood. They, too, are not based on any reasonable, logical thinking process but were blindly accepted as they were infused into the child's self-system by parents or significant others, school, society, and so on. The danger of values lies in their subconscious nature and lack of the person's awareness of the process, of their formation or their application in everyday situations.

As an example, a community health nurse may have grown up in a family that stressed orderliness and spent much time cleaning and tidying the house. As a young child the nurse has integrated her mother's message that a clean house is a sign of a good housewife and a good family. As a result of a natural thinking process, she has carried the concept a step further and concluded to herself that, if a clean house means good people, then an unclean house has to mean bad people. All through childhood she has not felt comfortable in homes where pots and pans were piled up in the kitchen or dirty clothes were strewn all over the living room. As a community nurse, the sight of a home that is untidy, according to her definition, creates within her a feeling of disgust, and consequently she separates herself emotionally from the people living in that home. Since the nurse expresses her feelings nonverbally, the client's family will sense some rejection and, as a result, a productive communication is not possible.

Even though the severity of the reaction described in this example may be exaggerated, every nurse reacts to values one way or another, and it is of utmost importance that community health nurses increase their awareness of such interference and stop it before it causes harm. Consequently, the first step leading to a productive interaction process is to recognize such gut feelings and quickly analyze where they come from before they interfere with nursing care.

It should be kept in mind that the client family may experience an equally severe reaction toward the nurse, especially if their previous experiences with the health care system have been disappointing. Ways to counteract or dampen such responses will be discussed later in this chapter.

The best indicator of an initial reaction is the nurse's feeling upon entering the home. The nurse needs to react to it without getting overwhelmed by it. Anxiety and apprehension will be high in a novice; the shock of feeling out of place and helpless may paralyze the student. The danger of feeling different and of not wanting to get closer to the client is real, even in the case of a nurse who has done visits for many years, where anxiety is no longer important in determining behavior. Remarks such as, "This family is impossible to work with," "These people don't listen," "This family says yes to all I teach but then ends up doing the opposite," "These people are beyond help" are only too familiar in a visiting nurse agency. These are consequences of subtle dynamics starting out with the very first visit, and once they happen they are hard to reverse.

The first questions that need to be asked are, "How do I feel about this family?" "Do I get a warm feeling of being accepted or are the people so different that I feel out of place?" "Does this home look like anything I am used to?" If the initial reaction is positive, nurses usually experience an instant relief. They can then assume that the people they deal with accept them, since their values do not greatly differ. If the feeling is negative, they have to bear in mind that this can be due to several factors, each one of which can be conquered in its own right.

- Expectations
- Value interference
- Role insecurity
- Client's reaction to the nurse

Expectations

Expectations consist of a preconceived notion of what the home visit will be like. Preparing for the visit, the nurse has set goals for the client family. The family is expected to learn and respond openly to the nurse. Beginning students' expectations, in particular, are often ideal. A student might expect to find the client, a postsurgical obese lady who needs diet teaching, alone at home, waiting and ready for the student to teach her diet principles. On entering, however, the student may be shocked to find several visitors in the living room, a dog and three young children running and screaming, while the client is busy talking on the telephone. The student might then try to do her diet teaching anyway and find herself being ineffective and disappointed. An experienced practitioner, instead, would reassess the situation and possibly use the time for socialization and winning trust in order to set up a new appointment.

Such a situation can be avoided if a thorough assessment is made prior to the visit. The more factors that can be incorporated in the assessment— such as number of children and other people living in the family, occupations of family members, and leisure-time preferences of the clients— the more likely it is for the nurse to be realistic. If a meeting with a family member can be arranged prior to the first session, the best time for regular meetings can be worked out with the client. Also, during the assessment the visiting nurse may pick up cues pointing out psychological factors such as actual willingness of the client to have a visit, suspicions about health professionals, or anger and resentment directed at the health care system. The more experienced nurse will know how to compare such data with different situations she previously has been involved in and predict the new situation fairly accurately.

Example

Assessment: 68-year-old woman. Lives with husband, age 70.

Discharged from hospital three days prior to visit. Fell and broke her ankle, now wearing a full-length cast. May ambulate with a walker but has difficulties; uses wheelchair temporarily.

Very active in senior citizen's group; received nearly 100 get-well cards. Spends day visiting with people or watching soap operas on TV.

Did most housework prior to accident; has help once a week for cleaning. Husband does gardening, now also is doing housework.

All doors tested for width to see whether a wheelchair fits through them—no problem. Handle bar installed and stool in the shower.

Upon being called, husband was grumpy. Stated they did not need a visit, that he could manage things himself. He seemed to be the authority in the home.

Client was willing to have a visit but said that from 2:00 to 5:00 she would be watching TV and in the morning two people were visiting.

Purpose of the Visit: Assessment of safety of the home. Possible referral to a meal catering service.

Interpretation: Husband is supportive. Tries hard to meet wife's needs. Possibly has anger toward health professionals and feels threatened in his autonomy. Might be insecure about his care-giving abilities. Client enjoys company. Would probably enjoy a visit if it were not for her husband's negative attitude.

Conclusion: The couple needs to see that the visiting nurse cares. Husband needs to feel competent and to get support for his actions.

Action Plan:
1) Make several phone calls before setting up an appointment. Talk to both. Show interest in woman's and husband's daily activities. Ask how they manage. Comment to husband about his helpfulness and skills. Offer help in case of problems.
2) Set up an appointment; let client determine the time. Explain you might be able to offer some suggestions to make daily routine easier.

Resulting Expectations: Nurse will be treated rather coldly by husband. Wife will be reluctant to socialize until her husband feels comfortable with the visit. She might tell the nurse how busy she is having visitors.

After a cool initial reception, the visit turned out favorably. The husband responded well to praise of his efficiency and showed the nurse with pride how he had modified the home. The client was pleased with the visit, showed appreciation for the offer of help, and actually wanted to keep the nurse longer than scheduled.

Many factors in home visits cannot be anticipated, or some cues may be missed during the first meeting with the client. Sometimes the nurse is forced into a situation without being able to make a prior assessment. If the information is insufficient, a wise nurse will mentally rehearse how to cope with the worst possible situation; any situation better than the expected one, obviously, will be a relief. The novice student should not, however, let his or her imagination run loose and so become incapacitated with anxiety. Students should seek help from their instructors or supervisors as resource persons to help formulate realistic expectations, give reassurance, and be supportive by accompanying them on visits or making themselves available by phone in case of emergency.

The following safety measures are ones each student or visiting nurse should be aware of:

- Familiarize yourself with the area of your visit ahead of time. If it is an unsafe area, take another person along with you.

- Get sufficient information about your client in order to determine whether the visit is safe, especially with a client of the opposite sex.
- Keep in touch with your instructor or supervisor. Leave the address and phone number where you can be reached, as well as the exact time of your visit.
- Avoid night visits if at all possible.
- Do not carry valuables with you.
- Drive your car with all doors locked.
- Do not walk long distances. Park the car close to the home even if you risk a parking ticket.
- If using public transportation, arrange your visit at a time when traffic routes are well traveled.

Professional nurses often visit places in less than favorable conditions, but they should not forget that they have the right to refuse a visit if they feel threatened, that they may ask another person to accompany them in order to feel safe, and that they may leave a dangerous situation such as a domestic argument or a drinking party immediately. Nurses have to be aware of potential risks such as assault and violence, but at the same time they need to keep the reality of such a possibility within its proper perspective and not let anxiety about it incapacitate them.

Value Interference

Since values are an integral part of people's self-system, they determine behavior and emotional responses. As previously mentioned, values subconsciously lead us to categorize people: "good guys" are like us, "bad guys" are not. Since the value system is strong and inflexible, a person reacts to another person exhibiting conflicting values with dislike and tries to keep a distance, sensing that interaction might lead to an argument. To counteract natural reactions to conflicting values is one of the greatest challenges in the health professions. Nurses have to learn to be tolerant and to accept people as they are. This is easier in a hospital situation, in which patients are partly stripped of their identity. Even though age, sex, and racial factors are still apparent in clients all dressed in identical hospital gowns and lying in identical beds, other factors such as clothes or living quarters, which could ordinarily evoke value-based responses, are removed. However, even in the sterile atmosphere of a hospital, all patients do not get equal treatment. The nurse's approach differs for those in the general ward and those in private rooms, for those with private physicians and those admitted through the clinic, for those recuperating from minor surgery and those dying from a terminal illness. Part of the contrast in approach is justified by a difference in needs these clients present: a significant part, however, is likely to be based on the nurse's value system. People working in hospitals know that news such as "Patient X has been in a mental institution," "Patient Y is a homosexual," or "Patient Z had three medical abortions" travels rapidly. As a result, nursing care is likely to change in terms of time spent with and empathy given to the client, time lapse before the patient's call-light is answered, and so on. A community nurse does not need to look for differences in looks, behavior, or lifestyle, and at times will need to exercise acute self-awareness and self-control, which in turn requires genuine love of humanity by which his or her motivation is continuously replenished. Values are emotional and have little to do with the rational, thinking part of our mind. But the rational mind can be employed to counteract negative impressions left by differing values.

The principle nurses have to remind themselves of at all times is that *all behavior has a purpose.* There are reasons why some people drink, lie, steal, or beat their children. Behavior is adaptive; it is an attempt to fulfill a need. At the same time, society sets norms that define different behaviors as acceptable or not. Social norms are not always congruent with individual needs to resort to certain behaviors in order to maintain an emotional balance. A man may, for example, have a tremendous amount of hostility owing to injustice and frustration and as a result may lose control and become abusive to his wife or children. The act serves as a tension release, but of course it is condemned by society and of course the community nurse cannot accept such behavior. However, in contrast to the general public, the nurse's attitude toward the violent person has to be accepting rather than punitive—accepting not of the behavior but of the person, whose defenses were paralyzed by excessive stress and unfulfilled needs. Health workers have to realize that they, too, have been inoculated with society's norms and that they need to retrain themselves to develop tolerance and understanding of people's problems.

As mentioned, if nurses are overcome by negative feelings upon entering a home, client families will sense this immediately; they will not open up to them with their real problems and feelings but rather treat them as intruders. Nurses should learn to brush off the first shock and become quickly able to show real concern. Rather than condemn unusual behavior, they should show interest and ask questions in order to understand it better: "What makes this person feel and act the way he does?" "Does the behavior have undesirable results?" "Is a change needed?" "If so, does the person also feel that a change is needed?"

Example

You visit Monica, an 18-year-old mother, whose nine-month-old baby lies in a bassinet smelling of urine, her expression a blank stare. The baby does not smile but turns her face away from yours. The apartment is dirty: dishes are piled high around the kitchen sink, the floors are covered with food particles and grease, overflowing laundry baskets are standing along the wall, and two dirty diapers lie under the kitchen table. Monica sits on the couch, brooding. The baby whimpers.

First reaction: This mother is neglecting her child. She does nothing. Even though she has nothing to do all day, she does not even keep her house clean. You are angry with her. How can she let herself go like this? Doesn't she have any sense of responsibility? This baby needs a mother!

Second thought: This mother's behavior has to be due to some problems you know nothing about but have to find out about. She looks depressed and preoccupied. She let you in because she probably wants help. You have to intervene and take care of her; only then will she take care of her baby.

The steps to overcome value judgments in this example are as follows:

- Listen to yourself; recognize your gut feelings.
- Remember that your emotions are not rational.
- Realize that all behavior has a purpose and that you cannot judge a situation until you know the details.
- Think of the person exhibiting aberrant behavior as the one who needs your help.
- Get interested in assessing that person's needs.

At times, a nurse realizes that acceptance of a certain situation or of certain values is not possible. Under such circumstances, it is best to recognize these limitations and arrange for someone else to take care of the family.

Role Insecurity

Another source of anxiety inexperienced community nurses feel upon entering a home is insecurity about the role they are expected to perform. People use several roles—role clusters—and the more practice they get in playing these roles, the more comfortable they feel (Duval 1977: 117). Children grow up playing the dependent role of son or daughter. During adolescence, when they are expected gradually to separate from their families and make decisions of their own, the stress produced by change in role is called role strain. Nursing, too, is a role one plays along with many others, such as student, roommate, or choir member. Nursing expects certain behavior from practitioners and the education process trains students to perform the role. Patients expect nurses to be friendly, helpful, diligent, and quick, and the nurse attempts to live up to their expectations. At the same time, the student works hard to fulfill the instructor's expectations as well as those of the head nurses and doctors on the unit. Every clinical setting requires adjustment, and time is needed until a novice feels comfortable.

Adjustment to the role of visiting nurse is especially difficult. The physical setting the community nurse needs to feel comfortable with is much more complex than that of a clinic or a hospital. With each home visit the nurse has to fit into a new environment and perform a different role, and the possibility of rehearsing the role ahead of time is limited. If the setting is similar to what they are used to, nurses feel more comfortable because they assume that the role they performed in other settings will be accepted by the present client family. If the setting represents different values, they might find themselves not knowing what role to act or find the family does not respond to their usual role positively, since their expectations are different.

The experienced nurse practices an assortment of roles, and selection of the most suitable role for a certain set of circumstances is no longer a conscious process but rather is based on a quick assessment of the client's needs.

Even the novice need not feel totally lost, however, since exposure to different roles is not limited to the nursing field. Experiences with siblings and friends' families may make one comfortable with children. Taking care of grandparents may make one aware of the needs of old people. Everyone has a rich selection of experiences and resources to draw from to help function in home visits.

In addition, any insecurity can be relieved if the novice simply listens to the client. If the family's ideas as to what is expected from the nurse do not correspond to what the nurse can offer, this can be clarified and left for the clients to decide whether they want to proceed or not.

Using the above methods can reduce basic anxiety so that a visiting nurse can better function in many different situations, although he or she will need to go through a period of testing, trying out different approaches and listening carefully to the client's feedback. Suppose, however, the shock of role insecurity is such that, despite these measures, the nurse loses self-confidence and is overwhelmed with anxiety. How can it be counteracted?

Anxiety, which is comparable to stage fright, varies with individual personality. Certain people are affected by it more than others, and some never quite outgrow it, even though their experience is extensive. Anxiety is mainly based on fears about the unknown: What will happen? What will these people think of me? What if they ask questions I cannot answer? Thus, eliminating as many unknowns as possible will decrease the anxiety. The student plagued by anxiety does better by meeting the client beforehand in a clinic, by looking up the home and doing a thorough assessment prior to the visit, or by doing a mental rehearsal of the role to be played during the visit. In addition, students should talk about their anxiety with an instructor or advisor, and, since anxiety is contagious, should avoid the company of other apprehensive students before a home visit and instead seek reassurance from those who have made visits. Indeed, asking such veterans to help formulate realistic expectations can be more reassuring even than talking with an instructor, since these are peers who have just lived through the same agony.

During the visit, students may want to employ relaxation techniques similar to those they use during stressful exams, such as breathing deeply, giving themselves pep talks, or picturing themselves floating through the air. Anxiety should be accepted as being helpful to a certain extent, since it activates one's capacity to think and perform; however, too much anxiety causes the opposite result, so its level should be monitored carefully.

Self-confidence can be further gained by realizing that one has probably mastered difficult situations on other occasions and that all these experiences from the past will help one cope with the present situation as well. It also helps to remember that many emotions felt in response to the client's verbal and nonverbal behavior are based on the student's value system and are not rational on many occasions but can and need to be controlled simply by understanding what is going on.

In summary, it is possible for a reasonably well adjusted student to control excessive anxiety and gain enough self-confidence by collecting as much information as possible about the client, the family, and the community they live in, so that expectations may be fairly realistic. This preliminary assessment process eliminates some of the unknown factors and allows the student mentally to rehearse the visit with more accuracy.

A student with such mental preparation who has a good background in communication techniques will likely have the flexibility to act appropriately even if unforeseen happenings occur, as the following example makes plain.

Example

Mr. Hoft, 56, has broken his lower leg and is now at home in a full-leg cast. During hospitalization a week ago, he was found to be hypokalemic from diuretics and blood-pressure medication. The nursing student, Dan, has planned a visit to Mr. Hoft's home to teach necessary diet changes that include high-potassium foods.

Upon entering, he finds Mr. Hoft has been running a fever for two days and has pain in the fracture site. Three days earlier he fell on the stairs to the backyard and cracked his cast above the ankle; the crack is covered with masking tape. He complains of pressure on the foot and he and his wife are worried; however, they did not call the doctor because of reluctance "to disturb such a busy man."

Dan's initial reaction is a sequence of panicky thoughts. This sounds like an emergency situation, and he has never dealt with similar circumstances. What to do? He recognizes, however, that high anxiety leads nowhere and that these people need his help. Taking a deep breath, he says, "It seems that before we talk about diet, we need to make sure your leg is okay. Tell me a little more about your accident." While Mr. Hoft tells him the story, he has time to think, integrate the information he hears, and formulate an action plan.

Dan then takes Mr. Hoft's temperature (99.2°) and blood pressure (110/60) and assesses the status of the injured leg. Although the toes are warm and pink and no stains are evident on the cast over the fracture site, Dan feels the temperature and Mr. Hoft's complaint of pressure on the leg warrant a visit with the doctor. He makes an appointment at the emergency room in two hours. Mr. Hoft being unable to concentrate on diet teaching, a second visit is scheduled for that purpose.

This example shows that listening to the client as well as to his own reactions has helped the student take appropriate actions—namely, to relieve Mr. Hoft's fear something might be wrong with his foot and to obtain physical assessment data supporting that suspicion. Dan then rightfully concluded the client would not now be receptive to diet teaching and decided to come back later. The next visit will also give him another chance to see how Mr. Hoft is progressing and to assess safety features within the home.

Culture gaps, racial differences, severe handicaps, or mental illness may make the nurse feel inadequate, but such problems can be bridged if the nurse listens to the client's needs and adjusts his or her role accordingly. The nurse, being able to recognize and control intervening emotions, is now ready to engage in the actual interpersonal process during the first encounter with the client family.

NURSE-CLIENT INTERACTION: THE INITIATION PHASE

The nurse-client relationship is thought to occur in three phases. The first phase is the initiation phase, which has the aim of building a trusting relationship, with the qualities of mutual respect, concern, and empathy. The other two phases, the working phase and the termination phase, will be discussed in Chapter 9.

The length of the initiation phase varies. Sometimes a few words of greeting to the client are sufficient to create an atmosphere conducive to teaching. Frequently, however, the client is suspicious or preoccupied, and does not view the visiting nurse as a welcome guest. Although the initiation phase of a relationship may turn out to be extremely wearing, and require several visits, its successful resolution is a necessity for productivity in the working phase.

Usually students entering nursing choose the profession because they have a desire to help people. In some situations within community health nursing, however, this desire may be greatly taxed and may be stifled if it is not coupled with a strong self-concept. The role of student nurse is not easy, and every nursing student is plagued with insecurity. And, clearly, it is difficult for an insecure person rejected by the client family to pursue the relationship with the same empathy and personal involvement. But yet this is what the therapeutic relationship asks for.

Upon entering a home, the nurse must be aware of certain factors. First, the client should be expected to be mistrusting. The nurse needs to recognize that clients may consider nursing visits to be intrusive, impinging on the family's right for privacy. Tact is essential, and little things count. Asking whether shoes should be removed to protect the carpet, inquiring where the family would be most comfortable for the teaching session, and the like, may improve the first impression a client has of the nurse, shorten the initiation phase, and make the working phase more productive.

With certain families it is difficult to build trust, especially if there are racial or cultural differences. In addition, the family may mistrust the nurse because they mistrust the health care system in general, having had unhappy experiences with long waits in clinics and not getting their needs met or being blamed for not seeking help sooner. Experience may also have taught them that they fare best with people not of their own kind if they are nice to them but keep them at a distance; thus, they may agree to a home visit but later "forget" to be home. The resentment is not usually against the nurse, however, and indeed often they truly forget because the home visit has very little importance to them, compared to the rest of their worries, and does not fulfill their needs. Students often feel shattered on realizing that a client has invested so little energy in the visit and seems to avoid any kind of commitment, especially if the visit is important for the student.

An evasive family may also be testing the nurse, since a certain amount of testing always happens during the initiation phase. Just as the nurse observes the family closely, so do the clients observe every move the nurse makes, trying to pick up insecurity, arrogance, or belittling behavior. Not being at home is a way of testing the nurse's commitment. It may also satisfy some unconscious urge to control the nurse, since being able to make the nurse angry means that the client is in a position of power. The issue of power or autonomy is an extremely important one for people in that part of the population who feel at the mercy of society and with little power to change their fate.

Example

The natural reaction of a nurse to testing, game playing, and evasive behavior is withdrawal and anger. Nurses often say: "If they don't want me, why waste my time!" Such injured self-esteem happens at times even with experienced nurses. The following example shows a few ways of dealing with this reaction.

Sheila, age 21; her alcoholic husband; and her three children, ages 4, 3, and 1½, are a problem family well known in the community. Barbara, the community health nurse, had been trying to get Tony, the eldest boy, to attend a Head Start program at the school, but he had gone a few times and then had to quit because Sheila had not met the requirement of having him immunized. The problem is now acute since Tony will be ready for kindergarten in a few months. In addition, Sheila has become pregnant with her fourth child.

"Guess what, Sheila did it again!" Barbara told her colleagues. "I taught her every method of birth control. I made an appointment for her at the clinic to get a copper-7, and she missed that and she missed the next one!

What can you do with these people? She's certainly not fit to be a mother. And this new kid is another one you and I are going to pay for. Her husband hasn't worked since he got out of jail. Wonder how he gets any money!"

Ann, the next nurse put in charge of the case, was new to the agency. The family has no telephone, so she tried several times to visit them. Though no one ever opened the door, once it seemed as if the curtains had moved at a window. "Something must have really turned this family off," she finally decides. Remembering what Barbara had told the office, she thinks, "This family is angry about the community nurse trying to force them into getting the child vaccinated and the mother into using birth control. I wonder if Barbara ever listened to their problems. These shots could not have meant very much to them since they had to cope with a father being released from jail. They probably just couldn't face another problem and instead took the boy out of school. Could it be that the mother read Barbara's pushing her into using birth control as meaning the nurse didn't think she was a good parent? Barbara actually expressed that, and I'll bet her attitude showed in her nonverbal behavior."

If the cooperation of the family is destroyed, what is Ann to do? Somehow she must meet Sheila and talk to her very cautiously to try to establish trust. She tries twice more to visit them, each time leaving a note saying that she cared and wondered how Sheila's pregnancy was going. On the third time, she meets Sheila at the door, her youngest child hiding behind her upon seeing the nurse. The nurse and Sheila look at each other a few seconds, then Sheila says angrily, "I don't need anything" and shuts the door behind her.

Ann is shocked. Sheila's angry, hateful look disturbs her deeply. She feels like withdrawing; after all, Sheila has the right to be left alone if she wants.

For the next few days Ann digests her resentment and hurt feelings and shares them with her supervisor. Together they conclude that since Sheila and her family have many needs and since her reaction seems to be based on the previous community nurse's insensitive approach, they should give it another try.

Ann makes an agreement with the clinical specialist at the prenatal clinic to be informed when Sheila is admitted to the hospital to have her baby. On the second day postpartum, she goes to visit Sheila. She feels very nervous. What is she to do so Sheila will not reject her again? She tells herself that if it happens she need not take it personally, since it was not her Sheila is angry about. She realizes she really has nothing to lose, that their relationship can only get better.

When Ann enters the room, Sheila's face expresses surprise. There is no smile but no anger either. The tension is palpable. Though feeling weak and insecure, Ann forces a smile, then waits. Signs of a beginning smile on Sheila's face give her courage. "Remember me? I heard about your baby and came to congratulate you. I saw him in the nursery. He's such a healthy little fellow. How are you feeling?"

The tension disappears, and Sheila begins sharing her problems. During later visits the nurse is able to advise her on a birth control method without resistance.

This example shows that success came about through Ann's

- Dealing with own emotions;
- Explaining to herself why Sheila would probably react as she did;
- Counteracting her natural wish to withdraw;
- Drawing upon own resources and deep caring for people;
- Being persistent and letting Sheila know that she cared in spite of her rejection.

Trust was then established by her

- Successfully reading Sheila's nonverbal behavior;
- Expressing concern and caring through nonverbal and verbal behavior;
- first addressing something positive, something that made Sheila feel good;
- Expressing readiness to listen to Sheila's needs.

CONCLUSION

A nurse who passes through the initiation stage with ease is the nurse who is—as Rogers (1961: 50–55) states in a passage describing the helping relationship—strong enough as a person to be separate from the other and secure enough to let the client be different. The first encounter between the client and nurse needs to be a time when an attitude of acceptance, caring, and desire to help is transmitted to the client verbally and nonverbally. The client needs to know that the nurse is ready to listen, that he or she is open and eager to answer questions and help solve problems.

Self-confidence helps to overcome any insecurity that stems from the nurse's being different from the client. The self-confident nurse can concentrate on the client's needs without feeling self-conscious about what the client might think of him or her and can pick up clues about the client's family, past and present life, joys and problems. Once insecurity is removed the nurse can actually enjoy the differences and explore with a healthy curiosity the client's world, the physical world, and the world of feelings, which can lead to personal growth and rich experiences.

REFERENCES

Berne E: *Transactional Analysis in Psychotherapy.* New York, Grove Press, 1961.
Duvall EM: *Marriage and Family Development,* ed 5. Philadelphia, Lippincott, 1977.
Rogers CR: *On Becoming a Person.* Boston, Houghton Mifflin, 1961.
Sullivan HS: *The Interpersonal Theory of Psychiatry.* New York, Norton, 1953.

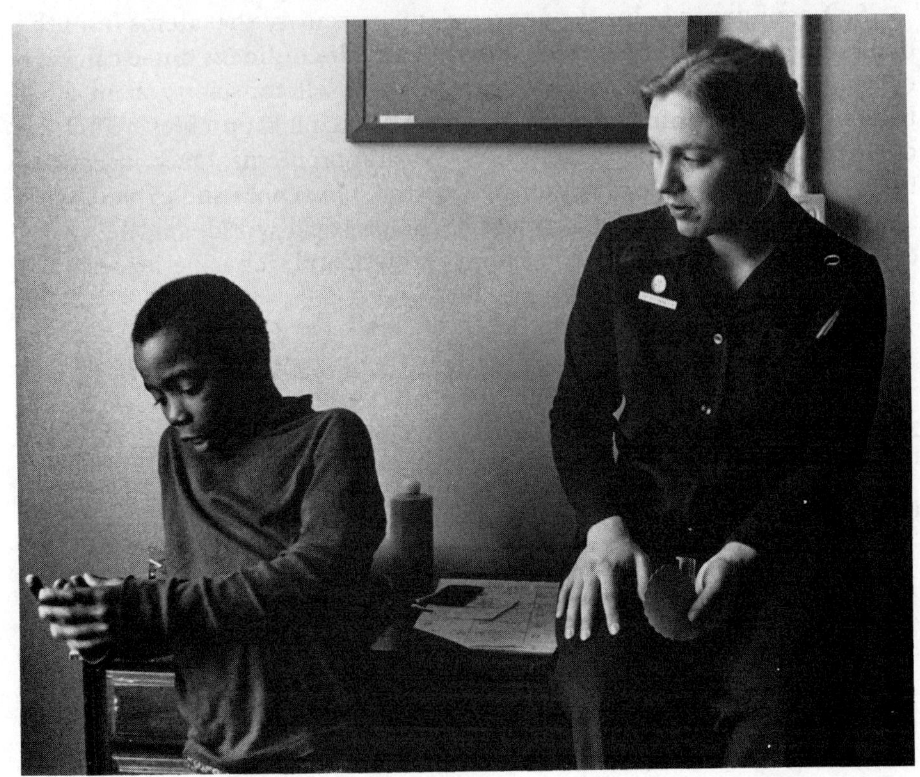

L. FLEESON/STOCK, BOSTON

8

Crisis Intervention in Community Health Nursing

Many practitioners in the health care field hold the common misconception that crisis intervention is a matter for the mental health field only. If that were true, the community health nurse would not have to be skilled in crisis intervention but would merely have to refer clients in crisis to a local crisis center and then retreat.

Crisis intervention, however, has become a model for practice in all health fields. The new type of intervention has been a reaction to the inefficiency of long-term psychotherapy with regard to solving acute problems. Self-help groups such as AA or Parents Anonymous seem to have risen as a result of people's unhappiness with professionals who tried to shape them into conforming to societal norms. Self-help or support groups are now available for clients for almost any kind of serious medical problems. Mastectomy clients find comfort in talking to women who have adjusted well to their loss, colostomy clients exchange experiences and ways of coping, parents of children with cancer unite to share their concerns and grief. At present, mental health crisis centers are largely staffed with volunteers who rely on their own personal experiences in dealing with the crises of clients. The message these people try to convey to the client is that they have lived through it and so the client can make it also.

This type of support is not new; indeed, it represents what nursing used to be, before it became "scientific." In the past, nursing was practiced by all concerned people in the community; people listened to each other's problems, pitched in when someone was in need of care, and organized self-help groups were nonexistent. Today, even though churches make an effort to recreate the atmosphere of concern and mutual assistance of people in times of trouble and pain, most members of the community are not part of such a support network. Their support system may be sufficient under normal circumstances, but when a crisis hits they find it difficult to cope. Consequently, self-help groups are needed in order for people to learn that it is all right to be different or that they are not alone with their troubles.

BACKGROUND FOR SUCCESSFUL CRISIS INTERVENTION

Although the self-help crisis approach is effective in many ways, it does not address any underlying determinants that might have led to the crisis. Often it encourages the client to be excessively dependent rather than to provide growth (Burgess, Baldwin 1981:11). Often, too, the crisis needs to be dealt with at a deeper level. Consequently, the belief that anyone can do crisis intervention and that no training is needed is erroneous. One should have not only the skills necessary for long-term therapy, such as for communication and for establishing a therapeutic relationship, but also the skills necessary for crisis intervention. A therapist needs to be perceptive, able to quickly understand problems, and capable of developing intervention strategies within a limited period of time. In implementing treatment strategies, the therapist needs to be able to find a balance between directing clients and simultaneously granting them autonomy to allow for growth.

According to Caplan (1964) and others, crisis intervention is not entirely present oriented but takes into account those aspects of the past that activated the crisis or might reactivate it again in the future. Consequently, it is also directed toward preventing a recurrence. The material assessed and used for intervention, however, is strictly limited to the crisis itself. The intervention focuses on reducing stress to a level at which the client can cope. The time frame of the intervention is short.

Success in crisis intervention is measured by the degree to which the client is again functioning at the pre-crisis level. Depending on the nature of crisis, the immediate intervention may be sufficient and no ongoing care will be needed. The crisis intervention may be a learning experience for the client that will help in future crises. If some past problem is detected and eliminated, reducing chances for further crisis, the intervention may be said to have been beneficial. Crisis intervention is thus a treatment in its own right.

How is crisis intervention related to community nursing? The approach suggested in Chapter 5 is an example of a nurse using crisis intervention. The nurse encounters a family with a client just discharged from the hospital. Family members are in crisis since they are insufficiently prepared and feel overwhelmed with their enormous responsibility. The preliminary assessment of the immediate needs of client and family and the quick strategic plan for teaching, which includes motivation and ability of the family as well as the actual implementation of the plan, are crisis interventions. The assessment excludes all the areas relevant for a primary prevention assessment except for the ones directly related to the client's care. Practical interventions are of utmost importance, instructing the family how to perform procedures. The aim is to get them to function, to make changes in time structuring, activity and rest patterns, division of labor, and so on. After these changes are made, they should perform efficiently and under the same level of stress as they did prior to the client's illness. If this aim is achieved, crisis intervention has been successful.

During subsequent visits, the community health nurse will continue doing crisis intervention by broadening the assessment to all areas of function. The nurse should also look for less obvious problems with client and family which might interfere with care and should evaluate the extent of adjustment that needs to be made. These visits, however, also include assessment and teaching in areas other than those related to the client's condition—for instance, a family member's pregnancy or obesity problem.

In most actual situations in community health nursing, crisis intervention constitutes only part of the intervention plan for a family. It is necessary that the community health nurse conceptualize the crisis. Even though an impulsive, empathic, and nonstructured approach to crisis may sometimes be therapeutic, most crisis situations require a structured intervention. The nurse needs to be highly aware of the dynamics of the crisis in order to intervene appropriately. Objectives have to be clear and precise so that time and energy are not wasted. As previously mentioned, during the refractory period the family needs help and support. The nurse should be involved in providing for their needs around the clock. Neighbors, friends, church members, and the like, may be mobilized to cook meals, watch children, drive them to appointments, and so on.

At the time patients develop awareness, emotional support is needed. No action is necessary at this point, but the nurse should give them permission to cry or scream if they need to and later to talk. The nurse should listen and convey a sense of deep concern and empathy. Often nurses feel uncomfortable in this role because they have been trained to *do* something about problems. Their feelings of powerlessness may remind them of unpleasant situations they previously experienced. However, nurses should realize that no analytical or technical skills are needed at this time and that their mere presence is a tremendous comfort to a family, although nurses themselves will invariably go through some emotional turmoil since they cannot help but identify with the family. Support is a true indication of caring and concern to the family, and it has a lasting effect on the relationship between nurse and family. The gratification resulting from it may be greater than that based on any other nursing intervention.

Nevertheless, the nurse should move cautiously in such highly emotional situations. An assessment should be made as to whether the nurse's support is actually needed. If other family members or close friends are present that the family feels closer to than to the nurse, and if they are giving necessary support, the nurse should accept this and tactfully leave. In such cases, a visit will be more appropriate at a later time.

Whereas the practical approach to crisis intervention can be a problem-solving process, we need to explore the underlying emotional dynamics. Let us look at four examples.

CRISES CAUSED BY SUDDEN EXTERNAL STRESS

The above described situation of the client discharged from the hospital belongs in this category. The affected person's trauma consists of the disease and the impact on the OLOF. The family feels the external stress of care giving. Families affected by such crises are usually functioning satisfactorily but then are suddenly hit by a traumatic event, such as an accident, a death, or loss of a job and lack of financial security.

Immediately after the trauma, the family or individual affected is in a state of shock, perhaps an incapacitating shock that renders usual coping techniques ineffective. This refractory period or time of emotional paralysis is a protective mechanism to prevent the stress-adaptation system from being overloaded. Since during this period the client or family is unable to make important decisions, draw conclusions, or engage in any kind of goal-directed activity, the main task of the nurse is to give support and make sure the family's needs are taken care of until its members are again functioning independently.

A traumatic experience, even if it does not directly involve a death, is experienced as a loss. For instance, for the client, disease means a loss of health, a trauma to the self-image of the body. An assault leads to loss of trust, loss of faith. Once the client has experienced the period of shock and disbelief that follows a loss and comes to realize what has actually happened, he or she will demonstrate emotional turmoil, sadness, pain, helplessness, hostility, anxiety, and anger. The question "Why me?" will be acute, especially if the traumatic event seems totally senseless, as in rape cases.

Community nurses involved with a family struck by such a sudden trauma have to base their intervention on the state of their response. Awareness of their own emotions is of paramount importance, for their presence in the situation should be based on the client's needs only, not on the nurses' desire to help. Nurses also need to be strong enough to feel separate from the clients, yet empathy is necessary, and nothing is wrong with shedding some tears together with a client. Above all, the traumatic event should not incapacitate the nurse or influence the care of other families. Nurses who feel overwhelmed and are unable sufficiently to control their emotions need to share the experience with other professionals. They need to work sad feelings through in order to find out how much emotional involvement they can allow themselves. Every individual must set limits to his or her emotional involvement, and the tool for doing this is self-awareness, as the following example makes clear.

Example

Sandy is a nursing student getting her clinical experience in a hospital emergency room. One day Kristen, a 25-year-old single woman, is brought in after a sexual assault that left injuries in the genital area as well as a stab wound in the chest. The violent act, luckily, was interrupted by neighbors who had heard Kristen's screaming. In the hospital, Kristen was rather quiet, looked fearful, and hesitated to talk to anyone she did not know well.

Sandy anticipated that Kristen might have special needs upon going home, so she arranged for a home visit two days after her discharge. During the visit Kristen did not say much initially. Sandy's opening questions, such as "How are you doing?" and "When will you go back to work?", received only one-word answers. But Kristen kept looking at her with eyes wide open; they seemed to cry for help. After a long moment of silence, Sandy summoned her courage and said, "Kristen, what's bothering you?"

The response was overwhelming. Kristen broke down sobbing, uttering things like, "I am so scared," "I can't sleep," "I see him in my dreams," "He follows me everywhere," "Why did he do it to me?", "Will he get me again?", "They haven't caught him." She clung to Sandy like a child, and she instinctively stroked her hair. Speechless, her heart pounded in her throat, Sandy had no idea what would happen next and sat immobilized with anxiety.

After a time Kristen stopped talking and just cried quietly. Sandy was able to collect herself and think about what to do next. "Kristen," she asked, "do you have a friend close by?"

"You can't leave me," Kristen answered. "I need you. Stay with me!" She repeated this over and over.

"I'll stay with you some time," Sandy finally answered, "but then I need to go. You can't stay alone tonight. Can you think of anyone who might have you stay with them for a night or two?"

Kristen seemed to be able to think rationally at this point. She mentioned a few people but stated that no one knew what had happened and that she had not told anyone because she was afraid they would think it had been her fault. She was ashamed of what had happened.

Sandy summoned all the information she knew from Kristen's case and the reading she had previously done about rape. From recent research studies she had learned that rape victims, against all logical reasoning, need to feel responsible for the rape in order to gain control and feel that they will be able to prevent the event from recurring (Medea and Thompson, 1974). Sandy therefore refrained from telling Kristen that she certainly could not have helped it and that if it had not been she it would have been another woman. She then offered to call one of her friends' family and explain the situation to them. After a lot of hesitation, Kristen agreed. Arrangements were made for Kristen to spend the night in their house. Then Sandy called her instructor, who suggested that Kristen get counseling from the assault crisis center. Sandy called, and Kristen talked to a counselor and made an appointment for a session the next day.

When she returned home Sandy was still shaken and although exhausted was unable to sleep. She was also preoccupied, unable to do homework, and relived the incident over and over in her mind. She felt terribly sorry for Kristen and anger toward the assailant, the police for not catching him, the society for not caring more, and God for not doing anything. Indeed, it took her over a week to become her normal self again. She told the story to her colleagues and family, and doing this helped her to get some of her feelings out.

There was one lasting effect, however, with regard to her nursing care. She still enjoyed doing things for her clients, but she felt hesitant to get involved in any kind of emotional problems they might have had. She felt rather aloof, looking at them from a safe distance. Her instructor alerted her to the fact that she did not respond to clients when they expressed feelings in order to get the emotional support they needed.

Sandy's reaction is a common symptom of overinvolvement. It occurs when the nurse is unprepared to cope with certain situations. Preparation for crisis intervention is possible, however. Had Sandy thoroughly prepared herself as described in Chapter 6, acquired knowledge about the common reactions of rape victims, and mentally rehearsed her role before seeing Kristen, she might have better coped with her feelings. With the damage done, however, she has the more difficult task of undoing it. She needs to increase her self-awareness. She will have to get involved with clients and give them permission to express themselves emotionally. Initially she may have to push herself hard and overcome her anxiety. In order to protect herself, she may want to choose clients without great emotional problems. She must then train herself to listen for clues the clients might give her which tell that they are willing to express themselves and to respond to these clues rather than ignore them. (Chapter 9 describes this process in more detail.)

In situations such as the death of a family member, nurses often feel very insecure about what to say, which words to use. The only advice we can give here is: Be genuine. A nurse should feel to a certain extent with the client, and whatever is said should arise from the emotional climate the nurse has created. The response should be honest without self-conscious motive. The words themselves are less important than the nonverbal behavior that goes along with them. Many times the client will pick up what is meant, even if the nurse struggles for words, and sometimes grabbing a client's hand without saying anything is more effective than an elaborate sentence of condolence.

The last stage of the grieving process is the period of restitution during which members of the client's family adjust to the changes caused by the crisis and rebuild their lives. The nurse's task during this period is to help the client to acknowledge the changes and learn new ways of coping. This is a time when it is helpful to do an extended assessment in order to compare the situation prior to the crisis and the circumstances after the crisis. The assessment also contributes in making the client aware of previously employed methods of coping in order to recognize strengths he or she had in the past which might increase self-confidence in the present. The intervention process in this stage is identical to tertiary prevention teaching, as described in Chapter 6.

CRISES CAUSED BY DRASTIC CHANGES IN LIFE

Crises of this nature occur when a family experiences significant changes over which they may or may not have any control: the birth of a child, the last child starting school, children leaving home, career changes, the wife starting work, or retirement. Many families master these events without a crisis; they consider them challenges and take pride and joy in mastering them. The difference between families that have no difficulties coping and those that do seems to depend on two factors:

- Accuracy of anticipation
- Basic attitude in life

Families that go into crises over life changes are not able realistically to anticipate what life will be like after a change. The crisis is precipitated by disappointment about what the imagined change actually turns out to be. Couples that get married often belong in this group. Being in love and excitement over the upcoming marriage make it impossible for them to recognize reality, so they are unprepared for the negative aspects that invariably accompany married life. Even though experienced people tell them about hardships, they do not listen. They rationalize that they are different and that such problems will not happen to them. The crisis occurs when they recognize that the glamour is over and they realize that they have to put up with another human being who turned out much less ideal than anticipated, who has his or her own needs and demands and often very different opinions. Such dreamers, who expect the world to come to them and make them happy, do not perceive a need actively to go out and work on creating happiness through a sense of accomplishment and self-satisfaction.

Prevention of such crises actually should be started early in a person's life. Messages from mother to daughter that success in dating and finding the right marriage partner will lead to happiness are not easy to reverse. Even new values and attitudes in society stemming from the women's liberation movement can lead to disillusionment; a woman seeking employment and fulfillment outside the home may be disturbed by family friction if husband and children are not willing to cooperate. Educating people to realistically examine facets of life is within the community nurse's purview, particularly in regard to children, both at home and in school. School nurses or nurses who are parents of children in school should do their share in upgrading social studies in elementary school so that the child gets a clearer picture of what life is actually like. The notion that children should be protected from the harshness of life is still prevalent and is the most vicious enemy of true anticipatory guidance. The community nurse involved on the family level can be a model by involving children in serious discussion concerning the family's problems. Many families show great surprise about how much children actually understand and how they contribute, comfort, and take responsibility. Children need to be part of the family's happenings; they should not be spared the pain of knowledge about illness, unemployment, and so on, since they pick up tension within the family anyway. But when they observe adults getting irritable, starting arguments, and looking tired, if they are not informed about the roots of the problems happening to the family they may get confused and even blame themselves for making their parents angry. Families that do not share their worries with the children actually do them a great disfavor.

One of the community nurse's most important tasks is the teaching of open communication. Family members need to talk about how they feel, and open communication prevents crises in this area, as well as others. Anticipatory guidance for adults about to experience life changes should not be ruled out as impossible just because an individual's outlook is idealistic and he or she did not have a chance really to gain insight into life's unpleasant counterparts, although the teaching process is more difficult, since clients need to be led to see that there actually is a problem.

Intervention once the crisis has occurred is very similar to anticipatory guidance. Clients affected by a life-change crisis need support to gain back their emotional balance. By listening to their problems, the nurse permits them to let off steam and find the sense of security and assurance needed to start dealing with the problems on a rational level. The aim of the intervention is to provide an in-depth understanding of the dynamics affecting the family system and the individuals, of the nature of the changes and all aspects of life affected by them. Teaching also includes expectations as to how the crisis can be resolved.

Example

A couple with a newborn baby needs to know that it is not unusual for new mothers to be exhausted and overwhelmed. The new role is complex and requires much adjustment, which often takes time. The baby is demanding and, of course, in no way considers the parents' needs for rest. Stress often diminishes breast-milk supply during the first few days at home. Some babies adjust to day-night routine with difficulty. Colic usually resolves at three months. However, eventually a routine is established if no other problems are involved.

A nurse can offer comfort to the new parents by pointing out that many other people have the same problems and resolve it successfully, that certain things will get easier with time: the baby will sleep longer at night and will become less fussy; the mother's supply of breast milk will be established, and so on. They need to be helped in learning their new roles, given practical tips for baby care, comforted by having a telephone number to call if questions need answering, and above all taught how to enjoy the baby. The nurse should make them aware how the baby learns by studying their faces and eventually recognizing them, how the baby follows a bright object with its eyes, how it reacts to sound, how it needs to suck. By describing to the parents what kind of a person their baby is, the nurse can help them to look at it with more understanding, acceptance, and pride.

DEVELOPMENTAL CRISES

Crises of this nature result from interpersonal difficulties based on developmental issues that have not permitted a person to reach emotional maturity. Unresolved issues about identity, dependency, autonomy, or sex image are particularly evident within the family structure. Such issues lead to exaggerated needs that spouse or children are usually unable to meet, and so the family engages in elaborate schemes and games that cause friction and, in some cases, violent clashes.

As police know and community nurses should know, domestic fights are the most dangerous situations to interfere with. If the nurse should witness a violent domestic argument or even threat of violence, he or she should leave the scene immediately. No attempt should be made to calm down the belligerents, for often the uncontrollable rage of both partners gets transferred onto the intruder. The nurse should make a judgment based on the family history and underlying problems to decide whether or not the police need to be called. There should be no hesitation if a weapon is involved.

Community health nurses usually do not witness violent arguments. In most cases, partners who have heated arguments on a regular basis will make a conscious effort to control themselves in the presence of the nurse. In fact, they may disguise their difficulties so efficiently that the nurse may leave with the impression that the family relationships are ideal. Troubles are mostly disclosed when one of the partners is absent. If the nurse asks a question or two indicating she observed a certain unhappiness or anger in the family, it may release a flood of complaints about the injustice, rudeness, inconsideration, and so on, of the partner. The role of the community health nurse in such a situation is to listen and try mentally to fit the pieces together and grasp the dynamics of the underlying problems. He or she should ask questions to collect additional data needed for full understanding, keeping in mind that an account given by one partner is never objective and that both partners are reacting to needs that are not being met. The nurse should not take sides but listen to each person's problems, acknowledging the difficulties and suffering.

Example

The following example illustrates how a nurse might proceed to handle a developmental crisis. Marianne has asked the community mental health agency for help with her daughter's eating problems. Cindy is five years old, very thin and pale, and has been absent many days from school during the winter owing to colds. Her kindergarten teacher has expressed concern about her nutritional status. The nurse finds Marianne knowledgeable about nutrition and extremely concerned. Cindy is encouraged to eat good food, vegetables, fruit, and meats. The family does not buy junk food, and sugar consumption is moderate. As Marianne sees it, the problem is that Cindy simply does not eat enough. She is not hungry, especially when she has colds, which is through most of the winter.

The nurse is somewhat baffled by Cindy's appearance and sickly disposition, since children her age eat relatively small portions and her food as described by her mother is nutritious. Asking Cindy to show her favorite toys and tell her what she likes to do, the nurse finds Cindy unresponsive and serious. She asks her mother, "Is there something Cindy is unhappy about?"

"She's scared of her Dad," Marianne replies. "He beats her."

It develops the troubles started when Cindy was first born, when she turned out to be a girl instead of a boy, as her father had wanted. She was also small, and did not have much resistance, and as she grew older her father set high standards for her, becoming upset if she did not pronounce words right, expecting her to walk before she was ready (calling her a coward when she refused to let go of the chair she was holding on to), then started fussing about her eating, trying to stuff her with food and creating scenes at the dinner table.

"How did you respond to all this?" the nurse asked. Marianne answered that she tried to protect Cindy and tried to make up for the father's strictness by letting the child get by with much more than she normally would.

Potty training was another difficult area. Cindy's father would fly into a rage when she had dirty pants and gave her many spankings. When Marianne would then take her in her arms to quiet her down and tell her she loved her, her husband would get furious and use foul language; once he even hit her in the face, although he apologized and never did it again. Now Marianne tries to remove Cindy from situations that could cause problems, and feeds her before her father comes home, picks up her toys, and cleans her. She feels guilty about her lack of power to protect Cindy. However, she also seems to need her around to comfort her, and when she is in school Marianne feels lonely. Thus, she keeps Cindy home from school whenever she has a runny nose or complains of stomachaches, which happens frequently. Marianne gets blamed by her husband for babying the girl.

"He's a jealous man," Marianne says about her husband. "He wants to possess me. But I don't love him any more. In fact, sometimes I really hate him."

Before Cindy was born, the couple lived in a shaky equilibrium. Marianne's husband had conflicts regarding issues of power, autonomy, and sexual identity, which Marianne was able to resolve only by playing a subordinate role and giving him lots of attention. The dependence on her husband did not bother Marianne until Cindy came along. The baby represented a failure to her father, who had wanted a son, and also, he felt, stole Marianne's time, energy, and love from him. Mother and daughter had such a wonderful relationship that he felt left out, and so he expressed his anger at the child. This, however, not only victimized the child but also converted his wife into an enemy. Since she thereupon began being angry with him, he felt justified in lashing back at her. Of course, this did not bring any relief; though he was able to reestablish his position of power, he could no longer fulfill his other needs—for love, security, and self-esteem and the esteem of his wife. Sexual relations turned into a struggle for power and satisfied neither; as a result both were left with unfulfilled needs.

The nurse recognizes that great harm has been done and that correction of the crisis is no longer simple. The underlying currents need to be recognized by both partners and the developmental issues need to be resolved. The aim of the nurse in such a situation is to interpret the dynamics, in particular, pointing out the effects of both parents' behavior on Cindy. Arranging a joint session with both partners, she points out her understanding of the problem affecting the happiness of both, being extremely careful to respond to both partner's needs. No one is blamed; instead, the nurse emphasizes that their problems are a response to stresses they had not been able to cope with.

Referral to a mental health agency, which is what this situation warrants, is often rejected by a client family. If a nurse is able to present the problems in some detail and get cooperation in making changes, the family may become more enthusiastic after seeing that positive benefits may actually happen and may be more agreeable to a referral. For the nurse, working toward a referral requires patience, understanding, and persistence. Available services should be described to clients in detail and with enthusiasm. One tactic that may get the family to approve more readily is for the nurse to have a liaison person from the agency of the proposed referral visit the family along with the nurse.

The urgency of the referral depends on the family's situation. The choice, of course, rests with the family, unless the situation involves breaking the law. In Cindy's situation, the nurse needs to assess the extent of the child's beatings. Because most parents are less than honest in describing their disciplining methods, child abuse is difficult to prove if there is no visible evidence. Still, parents should be made aware of the law and the nurse's legal obligation to report any kind of child abuse, although this risks destroying the therapeutic relationship because the nurse will seem to be betraying the family by reporting them. The difference between acceptable spanking and child abuse is a fine line, and the decision to report or not to report is at times very hard to make. If there is physical evidence, however, there is no excuse for a nurse not making a report. In cases such as the above, the nurse may want to make his or her reporting conditional on the family's accepting a referral to a mental health agency.

In any case, to confront a family with such a threat is difficult, and the nurse needs to be convinced of the correctness of his or her action. The family should then be told, not in a threatening way, but in words that convey that the action is meant for their own good. They should be told that Protective Services will not try to punish them but find ways to help them. The nurse should offer continued support and help. In spite of all possible preparation, nurses taking this route have to anticipate anger and hostility of the parents.

CRISES RESULTING FROM SEVERE EMOTIONAL OR PSYCHIATRIC PROBLEMS

Crises of this nature may or may not be precipitated by an external event, but if such an event is involved, the person affected responds to it much more acutely than does the average individual. The reason for this is some underlying psychopathologic disorder, such as a depressive disorder, history of psychosis, or other impairment in judgment and functioning that prevents one from taking responsibility for meeting his or her own needs. Such crises may involve abuse of drugs or alcohol as well.

Crisis intervention in such situations is difficult because of the unpredictability of response patterns. The community nurses encountering such a crisis must primarily be concerned with the safety of the client. Sometimes a client can be talked to and calmed down to the point where he or she is cooperative enough to be admitted to a hospital; at other times more drastic measures such as medication or restraints are needed, and the nurse must procure any necessary help such as an ambulance. In addition, the nurse must support the family as much as the client.

To assess the situation, which in many cases may be nothing more than guesswork, the nurse needs briefly to question the family and others about the circumstances leading to the crisis as well as the client's usual conditions. The real value of the nurse in such situations is in coordination of services for the client and the family, arranging for action to be taken, and keeping everyone as calm as possible. If the nurse is the only health professional present, he or she may have to make life-saving decisions. Leadership skills, clear thinking under high stress, and extreme self-control are needed.

It should be noted that crises of extreme severity are rare in community nursing, and indeed a nurse may never encounter them. Until such a situation occurs, however, no nurse can be sure how he or she will function; it depends on the nurse's own coping mechanisms and previous practice in high-tension situations.

Example

The following example shows how one nurse dealt with a difficult situation. The Dicks family has called their community nurse, Norman, to come and help them, since they were not able to control their 18-year-old son, Steven, who has been acting strangely for two weeks. The past three days Steven locked himself in his room most of the time, refusing to talk to anyone and hardly eating. When he left the house, he did not tell anyone, and some neighbors saw him aimlessly wandering around in a park. Attempts by family members to get him to talk only made him angry; when it was suggested that somebody should be called who could help, he left the room and slammed the door.

Based on the information he received on the telephone, Norman was prepared to encounter a psychiatric emergency. He inquired whether there were any weapons in the house. The family denied it although they had not been able to search Steven's room. Norman decided to visit and asked a colleague, Bob, to accompany him in case of violent behavior. On the way to the home, the two nurses discussed the alternatives: they would try to talk to Steven and get him to accept help or they would have him committed to a mental institution if the family was willing.

At the Dicks' home, Steven was shut in his room, and the nurses talked to the family. In making an assessment, they asked about Steven's functioning before his breakdown and the cause of the change. It was brought out that, although a very intelligent student, Steven had been a loner all through his school years, and studied instead of socializing with peers; he did not date until the latter part of his senior year in high school. Steven also had never been communicative with his family. Although he did tell them about his academic successes, for which he was rewarded with money and verbal recognition, he did not share his troubles. The family knew that Steven dated a girl during the last few months but Steven would not respond to any questions about her and never brought her home to meet them. The family suspected that the reason for the crisis was that the girl had broken up with Steven. Steven had graduated from high school three months previously and had unsuccessfully looked for a job.

Norman summarized the situation for the family: Steven apparently had difficulties coping with major changes in his life, such as his graduation, job search, and particularly the girl friend's rejection, and found it hard to adapt since he did not share his feelings with others. His mental breakdown was due to his coping mechanisms collapsing from stress, and he would need psychiatric help. He might need medication to calm him and get him in a state of mind in which he could again function rationally. He would also need the help of a mental health professional to sort out his problems and make changes. Commitment to a mental hospital would be necessary in order to protect Steven from harming himself or others and in order to meet his physical needs. If he voluntarily came to a psychiatric emergency room to get a comprehensive evaluation, his condition might turn out to be controllable with less harsh measures.

The family agreed to try to talk to Steven. Asked who Steven trusted most, everyone agreed it was his father. Norman and the father discussed what could be said to get Steven to come out of his room and respond to an offer of help. It was agreed the father should tell him that the family was worried about him, that they could see Steven was suffering, and that they wanted to help. He should be assured he would not be harmed in any way.

The father went to Steven's door and talked to him in a quiet, reassuring voice. For 15 minutes, Steven did not respond at all and the father repeated the same assurances. Finally, Steven opened the door and came out. His body trembled with anxiety, and first he pulled back when his father tried to touch him. Continuing to talk quietly, the father explained who the two nurses were. After a half hour, Steven let his father put his hand on his shoulder and lead him to the nurses' car, which was to go to the psychiatric emergency room. Steven had understood that this was the best help for him.

Table 8-1 summarizes the points nurses should remember if faced with a crisis.

TABLE 8-1. POINTS NURSES SHOULD REMEMBER IF FACED WITH A CRISIS OF ANY TYPE

The nurse should support the family through the crisis.

Step 1. Assess type of crisis.

Step 2. Do crisis assessment:
  • Symptoms of crisis
  • Circumstances leading to crisis
  • Functioning of client or family before crisis
  • Factors in client's psychological makeup that led to crisis (may be done later, after intervention started)

Step 3. Choose intervention based on steps 1 and 2

Step 4. Evaluate intervention in terms of postcrisis level of functioning (evaluation should be done whether nurses decide to intervene independently or to use a referral)

Step 5. After immediate danger removed, priority given to prevention of further crises or tertiary prevention

REFERENCES

Burgess A W, Baldwin BA: *Crisis Intervention Theory and Practice: A Clinical Handbook.* Englewood Cliffs, N.J., Prentice-Hall, 1981.
Caplan G: *Principles of Preventive Psychiatry.* New York, Basic Books, 1964.
Medea A, Thompson K: *Against Rape.* New York, Farrar, Strauss & Giroux, 1974.

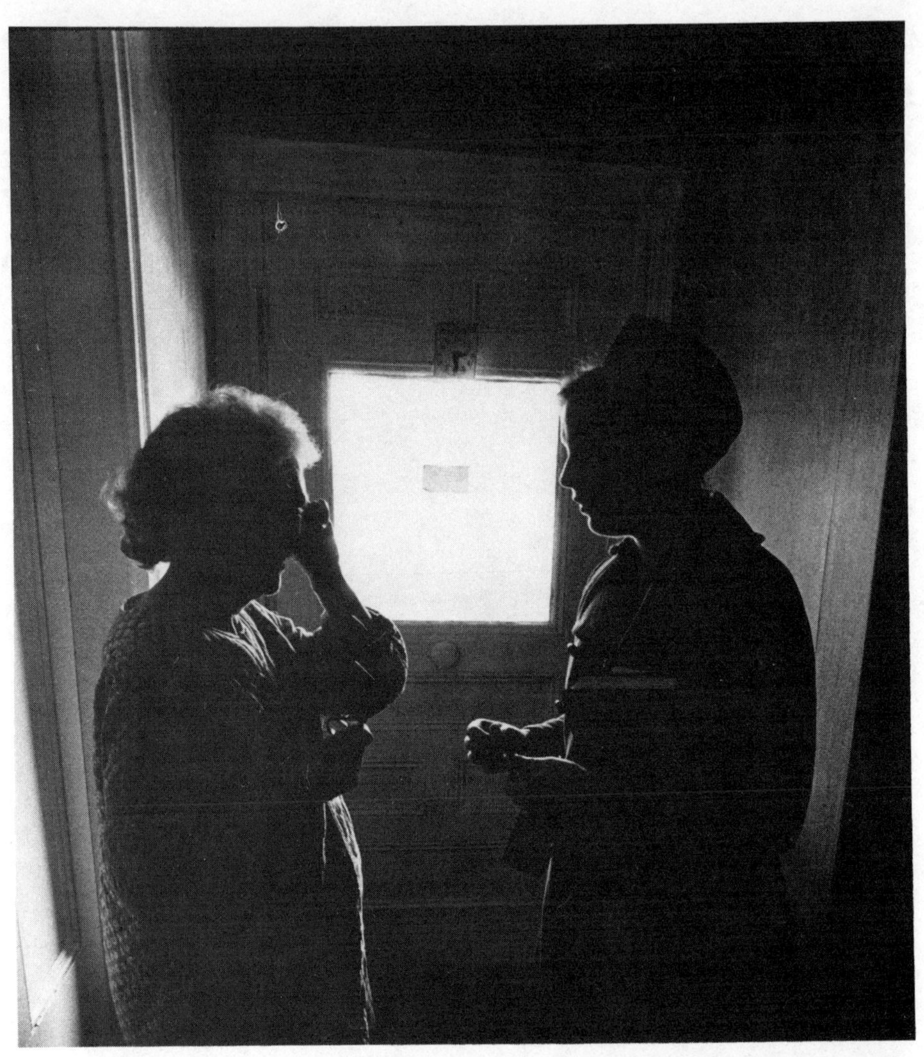

L. FLEESON/STOCK, BOSTON

9

Working with Clients:
The Importance of Communication

In Chapter 7 we discussed how communication is used to establish a relationship of trust. Chapter 8 showed that good communication is equally important in crisis intervention: The nurse must make quick decisions that under different circumstances would be deliberated at length with the family, yet their participation is of as great importance since the success of the restitution stage after the crisis will depend on the relationship the nurse has built with them. If competent action has led to respect and if the nurse has consciously included the family to preserve its dignity and its autonomy, a positive climate will have been created for an ongoing working relationship. On the other hand, if in the haste of action the nurse has overlooked the family's needs, some anger and resentment will be present later that will likely interfere with teaching.

COMMUNICATION IN THE WORKING RELATIONSHIP

Communication is the most important building block in the helping process, the problem-solving process, and the teaching process. We will not go into the theory of communication, which can be found in numerous books, but in this chapter will attempt to clarify its application to the nursing process. Nursing students should be mindful that studying the communication process may make them anxious or angry—anxious that, after memorizing all the techniques, nothing they say will be right or therapeutic, or angry that, after all the theory, a conversation will be so controlled and structured that it leaves no room for feelings. Students who find the communication process outlined in books foreign compared to what they have practiced in the past should not assume that their usual communication is wrong. Communication patterns should be left as they are unless the results they produce are not satisfactory. If a client reacts unfavorably to something that is said, the remark should be examined closely and consequently corrected.

However, there is indeed a danger that nurses will become so self-conscious as a result of studying communication techniques that they are no longer able to pick up the client's messages, nonverbal as well as verbal. A nursing student may go to and leave a client's house without ever noticing that the client looked tired from working long hours and staying up with a sick child and so was too preoccupied to really listen to the nurse's teaching. The real art of communication is not only the way messages are sent out, but also correct interpretation of messages received from the client. Every student should internalize the fact that listening is immensely more important than talking. An example will illustrate.

A nurse visited an elderly lady in a convalescent hospital. When she sat down next to her bed, the lady started telling her at length about the pain she was going through. Exhausting that subject, she recalled the good things in her life, including her family and children, and talked about the nurses in the hospital and little joys in her life. After a half hour, she said to the nurse, "This has been the best conversation I ever had. Thank you so much for coming!" The nurse had said barely a word the whole time. What had made the monologue into a "conversation," however, was the nurse's nonverbal messages to the client: *I really care. I understand your loneliness. I enjoy listening to your experiences and learning from them. You are a worthwhile human being.* Those messages were conveyed by eye contact, occasional smiles and nodding, and the warm touch of her hand.

Listening is a complex process. It is active and it is strenuous. It is the process of perceiving and integrating all nonverbal and verbal cues, finding patterns and discrepancies, and coming up with interpretations. The process is a team effort of all senses, rational thinking, and feelings. Consequently, listening in communication is not only hearing but *seeing* as well: observing for clues that tell the nurse whether the client actually means what he or she says or is sending out hidden messages, clues that let the nurse know whether the client trusts and respects him or her, expressions that reveal emotions the client may have but is reluctant to admit.

The ultimate aim of a conversation, other than the simple transmission of information, is to fulfill needs. Frequently, two people enjoy talking to each other not just because one person knows something that the other does not, but also because as they talk they reveal to each other aspects about themselves—and, if the partner reacts favorably, they feel good about themselves. In fact, the interpersonal psychosocial development theory stresses the importance of positive verbal and nonverbal feedback in shaping a person's ego (Sullivan, 1953). Since even a healthy ego needs regular positive reinforcement, communication is important for emotional health. Just as children invent all kinds of tricks to show off and be admired by adults, mature individuals use the communication process for the same purpose. Since society looks with disfavor on those who brag, individuals usually learn to disguise their motives skillfully. Such motives, the aim of which is to fulfill needs, become secondary motives within a conversation or lead to the playing of sometimes elaborate social games.

Most clients visited by community health nurses have in some way suffered either a blow or at least a threat to their egos owing to physical illness, high stress, or emotional difficulties. The nurse should therefore be well aware of their need to reinforce their self-esteem. The ability to pick up clues indicating such a desire may well mean the difference between a client trusting and liking the nurse or not. One easy way to detect these clues is to ask yourself the question, "Does the client talk on a rational level or on an emotional level?" Communication blocks can usually be avoided by responding on the same level.

Example:

  NURSE: Can you tell me what brought you to the hospital?

1. CLIENT: *(Sighs)* I had these terrific back pains. I didn't know what to do.

  NURSE: What did they turn out to be?

2. CLIENT: Kidney stones. *(Pause)*

  NURSE: When was your surgery?

3. CLIENT: Two days ago. I was so afraid, I thought I'd never make it out of here alive. *(Looks fearful, eyes wide open)*

  NURSE: But now that it's all over, aren't you glad?

4. CLIENT: Yes. *(Looks away)*

This nurse wanted to assess the client's history and was insensitive to the client's hints that she actually would have liked to tell the nurse how she felt. The client was looking for recognition of the anguish she had gone through in her first and third statements, but the nurse did not respond on the same emotional level. By looking away after the last statement the client conveyed that she felt rejected. Her feelings were very much part of her, and by the nurse's refusal to deal with them she felt personally rejected. An effective nurse would have responded as follows:

> NURSE: Can you tell what brought you to the hospital?

> 1. CLIENT: *(Sighs)* I had these terrific back pains. I didn't know what to do.

> NURSE: *(She thinks: She still looks all upset about it. It must have been a real shock for her. She probably was frightened thinking that she might be terminally ill. The nurse sits down and leans toward the client.)* Sounds like this was a real frightening experience for you.

> 2. CLIENT: Yes. You know, if you get these terrific pains out of the blue you start wondering. My mother died of liver cancer last year. Toward the end her pains were so bad she prayed to God to let her die.

> NURSE: *(She thinks: She sure had a lot of stress. It's understandable why she had trouble coping. She needs to know that I care. The nurse looks at the client compassionately.)* You had your share of pain, too, didn't you?

> 3. CLIENT: Yes, but the doctor said that the surgery went well and I will feel just like before or even better. Do you think he really meant it?

> NURSE: *(She thinks: She trusts me. She has some doubts, and she needs to hear from another person that she will be okay. She may feel better if I tell her exactly what was done so that she understands.)* I can see why you have some difficulties believing the good news. I'll go and find out the exact details of your surgery, then I'll come back and tell you. You can ask me any questions you like.

    4. CLIENT: Thank you! *(Big smile)*

The second nurse responded to the client's feelings; the actual communication technique used in the response is far less important than the fact that the client's needs were recognized and the secondary messages were interpreted correctly.

It is easier for a beginner to develop awareness of the client's level of communication, rational or emotional, than it is to pick the "right" communication technique among many within a fraction of a second. Being less anxious about the difficulty of answering therapeutically gives the nurse freedom to observe and feel with the client—in short, to listen to the client. If the nurse's genuine feelings are involved in the response, the client usually detects this and responds positively, even if the words the nurse has used were clumsy, since the significant communication happened nonverbally. Table 9-1 summarizes the significant steps in applying communication techniques in the nursing process.

"Levels of communication" are understood and explained differently by various authors. Transactional analysis (Berne 1961) sees verbal interactions happening on three levels, the Child (feeling level), the Parent

TABLE 9-1. APPLICATION OF COMMUNICATION TECHNIQUES

1. Observe the client for nonverbal behavior:
   - Gesture
   - Posture
   - Facial expression
   - Mode of speech
   - Eye contact, and so on

   What does the client seem to feel when talking?

2. Observe and listen for secondary messages: Does the client actually mean what he or she says? Does he or she want to express something other than the verbal message?

3. Based on 1 and 2 above, decide whether the client communicates on the rational or the emotional level and how he or she wants the nurse to respond.

4. Respond on the same level as the client:
   - Let empathy and concern be part of the response.
   - Do not be overly concerned with methods for a response—for example, restatement, exploring, clarifying, interpreting, summarizing—but know them and be aware of their effectiveness.
   - Avoid communication blocks—for example, false reassurance, stating one's opinion, jumping to conclusions, changing the subject.

(authoritative level), and the Adult (rational level). Powell (1969) explains communication by using five levels: Cliché conversation, reporting facts, sharing personal ideas and judgments, sharing feelings, and peak communication. These levels are distinguished by a difference in depth of the conversation and the person's willingness to share. For all practical purposes, thinking on two levels is easier, less confusing, and very effective. If trust has been established and if the nurse skillfully interprets the client's messages and responds to them, the conversation is likely to proceed through Powell's stages to the sharing level and, on some rare occasions, "peak communication" accompanied by a sense of "oneness."

The same process is helpful in handling silence. Rather than being overwhelmed by anxiety about the silence, the nurse makes a conscious effort to observe the client and analyze nonverbal behavior. This activity should lead to the conclusion whether the silence is beneficial, as is the case with the client who does mental problem solving during silences, or whether the silence should be interrupted. The client whose eyes wander, who looks out of the window, or who observes other people in the room may need to be brought back to the subject, whereas someone who is looking down, frowning, and giving the impression of thinking should be given the time to do so. During silences nurses need to be aware of their own emotions. In fact, this awareness is very much part of active listening. Silence creates anxiety. Insecure nurses fear that the client does not respond satisfactorily because he or she does not like them. The fear of rejection, which is a threat to their self-esteem, leads them to make doubly sure that the client knows what they mean. They interrupt silences and do not give the client time to think and reflect on what was previously said. Anxiety leads to being too talkative, too quick to respond, and negligent in assessing the client's messages.

Being aware of their own emotions not only helps nurses to control silences but also to control their level of involvement with the client, in order to avoid overidentification with the client and being overwhelmed in situations where the client becomes very emotional (as in the example of Sandy in Chapter 8). Some nurses are functioning at a high level of self-awareness, others are not. Nurses who need to train themselves can do so by writing a diary and thereby reliving the events of the day and the emotions that accompanied such events. Nurses who prefer not to write can practice verbal sharing with friends and family and through this process explore motives and feelings that led to certain behaviors. Participation in groups in which any kind of sharing is practiced is very helpful, and the person who needs special help should consider psychotherapy.

Self-awareness is the most valuable tool for communication in less than ideal situations. The situations community health nurses most often encounter are noncommunicative clients, clients who talk too much, manipulative clients, and clients with unpredictable behavior. In all four circumstances, nurses need to modify their usual approach. If their therapeutic process as a rule is nondirective in nature, these types of clients require more direction and guidance.

The Noncommunicative Client

Such clients are quiet persons. They may be withdrawn and preoccupied with their own world, they may be angry, or they may be very aware of what is going on but prefer to let others do the talking. When the nurse is doing a family visit, it is easy to overlook quiet family members, as probably most people who visit the family do. Quiet persons may not resent this, since they are used to it. Their needs, however, are no different from those of other people. They, too, need social interaction, and their self-esteem needs to be reinforced by people responding positively to them.

Confronted with a noncommunicative client, experienced nurses who have a fair amount of self-awareness recognize their feelings of uneasiness and natural urge to avoid the situation. Perceiving that their behavior may be nontherapeutic, they counteract it by going through the steps listed in Table 9-1 with heightened awareness.

Observing the noncommunicative patient is extremely important since in reality this client is communicating also, but on a nonverbal basis. Nonverbal communication gives some clues not only about how the client feels, but also about whether he or she likes the nurse or not. Signs of rejection naturally cause feelings of uneasiness and anxiety within the nurse, and again the impulse to retreat needs to be counteracted. Anger can have many roots. The client may have had bad experiences with health personnel, there might be a cultural prejudice, or the anger may be specifically directed at the individual nurse because of something that went wrong on a previous visit. Because such anger interferes with the therapeutic process, the nurse needs to confront the client with it, saying, for example, "You look angry today. Is there something I did that upset you?" The client may never admit that he or she found the nurse upsetting; however, the anger may subside from recognition that the nurse is concerned about his or her feelings. Such statements are hard to make owing to the fear that they might cause an angry outbreak from the client and threaten the nurse's integrity. In reality, this possibility is slim, and even if it occurs, it may relieve tension and lead to a better relationship. If the nurse can maintain self control and rational understanding of the situation, the case is usually won.

In case of withdrawn clients, the nurse needs first to draw their attention and stimulate them, so that they do communicate, either with a few words or nonverbally. When visiting a family for the first time, one way of getting the quiet person's attention is by the nurse's introducing himself or herself once more to the person, explaining the purpose of the visit, and making small talk. Extreme caution is necessary, however, to avoid belittling or talking down to the client. Since the client may suffer from low self-esteem initially, the nurse's attitude has to promote dignity and respect.

After observing the client's nonverbal behavior and response to the nurse's introductory statements, the nurse might say something such as, "Mr. B., you seem to enjoy reading your paper. Your armchair looks real comfortable" or, "Mrs. F., your thoughts must have been far away. Are you feeling lonely here?" Although the client may only nod or answer with one or two words and open-ended questions may be of no use, the communication needs to be made for the client, despite the fact that this is difficult when the nurse knows little about the client. Comments can be made about objects in the home, such as family photographs; often clients like to say things about people they are emotionally attached to. Once such a beginning has been made, it helps to start conversation on the next visit as well. The nurse can then ask if the client has had any news from the person they talked about last time. By and by the nurse will learn more about the client and have more subjects to talk about.

Any nurse dealing with a noncommunicative client, however, needs to be aware of the danger of falling into pattern of interrogation, in which the nurse is asking question after question while the client responds with one-word answers. The conversation led by the nurse needs to be directive, but questions need to be nonobtrusive and interspersed with observations the nurse had made. For example:

NURSE: Mr. W., look at your ankle. Can you see? It's puffy. *(The client looks down, but is silent.)* I'm concerned about it because it means that the circulation in your leg is not as it should be. Does the leg bother you?

CLIENT: No.

NURSE: But it gets big, especially when it's hot, right?

CLIENT: Yes. *(Looks with questioning eyes)*

NURSE: Would you like to know what to do about it?

CLIENT: Yes.

(The nurse then continues by telling him how to elevate the leg, and so forth.)

If clients are not visited individually but are part of a family group, the nurse has to make a conscious effort to pull them into the conversation by asking their opinions with simple questions, stressing their needs to other family members, or by commenting on observations of their nonverbal behavior—for example, "Mr. Z. does not look happy about this decision [to call a sitter]. Would you rather stay home alone for a couple of days, Mr. Z.?" When teaching an area that concerns the noncommunicative member, the teaching should be done directly to the concerned member, with the other members as onlookers, rather than to the other family members on the assumption that they will inform the noncommunicative member.

The Talkative Client

Visits with talkative clients can become frustrating for a community health nurse, particularly under time pressure. Such clients may have coffee and cookies ready for the nurse, so that a home visit that was to be 20 minutes in length turns out to take two hours and the nurse emerges with enough material on the client's history and daily activities to fill a book. The problem is not how to start a conversation but how to end it and how to keep the client on track.

Initially the nurse needs to structure the visit and set limits for the client, telling the client how much time is available for the visit and roughly what is to be achieved during that time. These guidelines are helpful when it becomes necessary later to remind the client to return to the essential topic that has not been covered and time is running short. Usually the client knows that being talkative is a problem and does not get upset if the nurse interrupts to put the conversation back on the right track.

At times, of course, it is hard to find even a pause or moment's silence in the client's speech, and the nurse may get anxious and angry about not being able to cover what was planned. At that point, recognizing those feelings, the nurse simply needs to interrupt and explain the problem or else the conversation will become nontherapeutic. Interruptions can be made without hurting the client's feelings if tactfully worded—for example, "Mrs. A., what you tell me is very interesting, but time flies and we still need to talk about your diet. Can you tell me what you had for a fruit exchange this morning?"

Open-ended questions have to be used with caution in communication with these types of clients, since they will elaborate endlessly on every question if the nurse gives them a chance. Being more directive means using more closed questions and on some occasions giving them a choice between answers rather than waiting for them to come up with solutions. For example, a nurse might say:

> *Mrs. A., I hear you say that you skip breakfast often, and you agree that this is a habit you would like to change. I can see two ways you could do that—either by changing your total meal schedule so that you eat breakfast later, about 11 A.M., lunch at 2 P.M., and dinner at 8 or 9 P.M., or you change your routine of the day by getting up earlier. Which seems easier to do for you?*

Such solutions should be carefully evaluated, however, before they are presented. They should be based on data the clients have previously provided and should include all their problems. If clients are presented with the solution, they have to see the solution as being in their best interests and not as something that was fabricated at random by the nurse. Again, in order to integrate information and arrive at personalized solutions, the nurse must listen actively.

The Manipulative Client

Manipulative clients use the nurse to fulfill a need and expect the nurse to perform some role that goes beyond the defined helping role. Manipulations often are subtle, and a nurse may fall for them because, by doing what clients ask for, the nurse's needs are taken care of as well. Once the nurse is sucked into a behavior pattern of this nature, it is hard to get out. A client may select "her special nurse" and keep telling the nurse how wonderful he or she is, how much better at doing her duty compared to other nurses, and so on. In exchange for that personal gratification, the client may ask the nurse to do little favors such as running errands or other demands clearly not within the job description of the nurse. The nurse may do the favors in order not to disappoint the client who is so good to him or her, but a relationship of this kind clearly is nontherapeutic. Eventually the client's demands will create resentment, and the nonassertive nurse will then visit less frequently or simply no longer listen to the client's real needs. The client is also likely to use this manipulative approach to get people to do things for her with friends and neighbors as well—and, of course, they too will distance themselves from her if they feel used, and the client will remain lonely and unhappy. The effective nurse will recognize this pattern, prevent it before it happens, and point it out to the client in order to work with him or her toward change.

The best quality a nurse needs to have to handle this type of client is assertiveness. The first step in any relationship is to define the role. If this is clearly done, the client can be effectively reminded of what has been previously discussed. Manipulative clients need limits set. They need to have certain rules spelled out for them which other clients accept for granted. They need to know that a nurse is not "their" nurse but that each nurse has many clients and does not favor any of them. Male patients with female nurses often need to be reminded that the nurses' caring stems from feelings of concern and not sexual motives. Clients who use their "pretty little student nurse" to brag to their friends need to be confronted with their behavior.

The nurse's emotional reaction should be the indicator. Anger and resentment toward the client's behavior suggests strongly that change in the relationship is needed. The situation has to be openly discussed with the client. The nurse needs to alert the client to the fact that the manipulative behavior is affecting the relationship. When confronting the client three points need to be stressed:

1.   The nurse needs to recognize that the client's behavior has a purpose. Its root is most likely an unfulfilled need.

2.   The nurse does *not* transmit anger and resentment onto the client. Personal emotions need to be under control.

3.   The nurse stresses that only the client's behavior is not acceptable. The client still needs to feel accepted as a person.

Once the client is ready to work on changing the relationship, a redefinition of the nurse's role is necessary and limits are discussed and agreed upon by the client and the nurse.

Dishonesty, if discovered by the nurse, is handled much the same way. When discovering that the client has been lying, a nurse might react with a strong feeling of being betrayed. Such a feeling is particularly prominent if the nurse has made a strong emotional commitment toward helping this client. Confronting the client can consequently take the turn of punitive action, where nurses put themselves into the power position and look at the client much like a naughty child. Clients who resort to dishonesty do so for psychological reasons and their self-esteem is low as a rule. A therapeutic communication should therefore have the aim of strengthening their self-esteem rather than weakening it even further. Nurses need firmly to control their impulses and proceed through the same steps as with any other kind of manipulative behavior.

The Unpredictable Client

People's behavior is usually predictable to some extent, since culture determines how people relate to each other and respond to each other. Culture has trained people to send messages in a certain way in order to be understood. If it was not for these unwritten rules and patterns, communication would be practically impossible.

In order for communication to serve as a tool for mutual understanding, learning and teaching, it needs to be understood by both parties. When the nurse sends out messages, they need to be interpreted correctly by the client and vice versa. As previously discussed, factors that may distort the interpretation of such messages are emotional factors that interfere with the active listening process. Physical factors, such as tiredness or deafness, as well as intellectual factors at times prevent messages from being received correctly. The last group of factors which distort communication are the social or psychiatric factors.

Social factors are those determined by difference in culture, language, ethnic background, or status. Psychiatric factors are the differences in perception and behavioral responses of psychiatric clients compared to the average person. These last groups of factors are anxiety producing for the nurse who is unfamiliar with such clients and therefore unable to predict their behavior and their response to communication messages.

Anxiety of the nurse may be an even more significant factor in disturbing communication than ethnic differences or psychiatric disorders. Nurses feel most comfortable with their own kind of people. Anxiety consists of not knowing what will happen as a result of what the nurse states. The big question is whether the family will accept or reject the nurse and what needs to be said to assure acceptance.

Initially the nurse needs to spend time getting to know the family and their behavior patterns or the psychiatric client. Behavior is not totally unpredictable. Even severely mentally ill clients' behavior has patterns:

certain things will irritate them, others will calm them down. The pattern may be highly individualistic, so the nurse needs to learn to communicate in a specific way with each mentally ill client.

Families from another culture should pose less of a threat to the nurse. Certain ways of communication are universally human and understood. A smile, for example, tells the family that the nurse accepts them. If the nurse attempts to communicate in a foreign language, even if the conversation is not eloquent, the family unmistakably appreciates the effort and considers it a sign that the nurse truly cares.

Books are helpful sources of knowledge about different cultures which the nurse may find helpful, and this knowledge should be applied. For example, in Chinese culture, old people have respect and authority, and the young consult them for advice. Thus, a nurse would be wise to include grandmother who lives two blocks away when teaching a Chinese family about diet or birth control. Although grandmother may be harder to convince of the validity of new concepts, as long as she does not agree, the younger members of the family will not change their pattern either.

In the United States, families of foreign origin in certain ways adhere to their original culture but also adapt differently to the new culture. The community nurse should consider it a challenge rather than a threat to learn about different customs, life patterns, and values. He or she needs to listen and learn and refrain from giving advice based on the nurse's values rather than the client's. Communication becomes easier if the nurse is able to show interest and respects the family for being different.

Certain families are difficult to approach since they fear intrusion and are suspicious toward strangers. As in the example of Sheila in Chapter 7, the nurse needs a certain amount of ingenuity to gain access to the family. Whatever technique is used, once the nurse is allowed in, he or she should remember the following points:

1.   Be friendly and show interest in the family, the home, certain objects, the children.

2.   Avoid excessive behavior such as loud laughing, very serious expression, talkativeness, arrogance, humor.

3.   Observe and listen to what is said and done. Ask questions about cultural practices.

4.   Avoid stereotyping. Verify impressions about the family by discussing them with the family.

5.   Analyze how cultural practices and lifestyles influence nursing care and teaching.

6.   Adapt the care to the family's values.

These points are valid to a certain extent for psychiatric patients, the mentally retarded, or any person who is different in one way or another. Here, too, the nurse needs to proceed cautiously by avoiding excessive behavior. The nurse should allow time to get to know the client and should point out positive aspects observed about the client. Any praise must be meant honestly, however, since even mentally impaired people are as a rule quite skilled in detecting dishonesty. If the nurse listens to and shows interest in and respect for the client, the mentally ill or impaired person often responds positively. In fact, caution has to be used to prevent excessive dependency on the part of a person who usually fails to get respect from other people.

The Child

Community health nurses who visit families with children often neglect to include the children in discussions. They may say a few words to them and then ignore them except when they turn out to be disruptive, which invariably happens if no attention is paid to them. A child should be made part of the family-nurse group. Infants, if awake, should be held and cuddled by the parents or the nurse and talked to and stimulated. Toddlers also usually like physical touching and may want to sit on the nurse's lap, explore the medical equipment, and need to be talked to and given something to do. Older children can be communicated with through play; they should be given the opportunity to participate in learning about primary prevention, which the nurse can demonstrate with pictures, models, role playing, and so on, since children learn by doing. Often the adults too welcome change and their learning is reinforced if the nurse can, for example, do a role-playing act about nutrition. This can be made special fun for all if, for instance, the roles are reversed and the father plays a little boy who does not like vegetables.

All such games have to be adapted to children's ages and character and their ability to participate. The outgoing child will enjoy role playing, puppets, and imaginary play with dolls and objects. The quiet child may play with dolls too but may not communicate the events verbally, may take longer to warm up, and may want picture books to stimulate the sharing of thoughts and feelings. Drawing is another excellent way to let children communicate; if the nurse admires their art work, they will usually give an interpretation that may well lead into a conversation.

Ideally, the children should learn what the adults learn at the same time the adults learn it but with limited depth and understanding. If the children's interests are awakened, they will later stimulate the adults by their questions. In conversing with children of all ages, nurses should keep in mind the following:

1. They should be talked to in proper language. They need correct verbal stimulation for language learning. Children addressed in baby talk by a nurse, if they are not used to it, feel offended.

2. The nurse needs to be honest in all respects. Children will feel betrayed if a nurse says that a procedure will not hurt and then it actually does hurt.

3. Children's logic is not the same as the adults'. Children draw conclusions that are absurd to an adult. They see relationships adults would never see; for example, because Johnny's grandmother cut her finger in the kitchen at the same time he was eating an apple, Johnny may now refuse to eat apples because he does not want Grandma to bleed.

4. The nurse needs to explore how children understand certain phenomena and clear up misconceptions (see point 3).

5. Children are egocentric, and communication has to be directly concerned with them. When the nurse is teaching children, they need to know how the material being taught affects them.

6. If children are to do something, they should be told so firmly. They should not be given a choice if there is none, and they should not be bribed or promised something. The child older than age two needs to be given a reason why he or she needs to do it.

7. Children's feelings should be respected. They should not be told not to cry or not to be angry. However, they should be told how their behavior affects the nurse—for example, "I keep telling you that you cannot have this, but you take it anyway. That makes me angry!"

8. Children need firm limits. If the parents are inconsistent, the nurse should persistently reinforce limits and act as a role model to the parents. Children should be told exactly what is expected of them.

The talent to understand and converse with children varies among nurses. Experience has much to do with the ingenuity of approach and the success of being accepted by the children. Unless the nurse has a personal problem, there is no reason why even the inexperienced nurse cannot learn to be successful with children. At times, nurses fear children's undisguised honesty and their rejection. They should keep in mind, however, that such judgments usually occur on the spur of the moment.

If young children say "I hate you" either they are angry at the nurse momentarily or they want to test the nurse. Being able to make someone feel bad provides children with a great sense of power. At the same time, if that person likes them in spite of what they said, it means unconditional liking, and that is what they want. Children are excellent observers of nonverbal behavior. After saying "I hate you," they will closely observe the nurse's reaction and then form an opinion about what kind of person the nurse is. A nurse who dislikes children will not be liked by them; one who likes them will be forgiven many blunders of communication without losing their trust.

Nurses grow to like children by getting used to them. Babysitting or volunteering in a day-care center are excellent opportunities for nurses who need the experience.

Teenagers have different needs. Since they are working on separation from their parents, it is often preferable to have individual sessions with them rather than including them in family discussions. Many adolescents do well in groups. Teaching of areas that concern teenagers should be done in groups, with sharing among peers encouraged. Within family sessions, the adolescent should be allowed to listen quietly, if he or she chooses to do so, without being pressured to speak up. Honesty and genuineness of expression and feelings are extremely important in communicating with teenagers.

THE HELPING RELATIONSHIP

The principles discussed so far in Chapters 7–9 are practically inseparable from the helping relationship concept. The helping relationship, which is formed in the initial contact with a family or individual, is used in crisis intervention, problem solving with clients, or in teaching. The helping relationship is not unique to nursing, being practiced also by ministers, social workers, doctors, teachers, and parents. It occurs whenever one person has a need and another person helps to meet that need.

Interaction within a helping relationship is somewhat different from that within a social relationship. In the social relationship the roles of the participants are equal; in the helping process, there is a helper and a client with a need. Though both parties contribute to the process, the helper is the leader. Interaction between the parties is structured, goal oriented, and more intense than in a social relationship. In the helping relationship, the focus is on significant personal issues and the helper is required to have acute self-knowledge. In the social relationship, issues are superficial and participants maintain a safe distance from and sense of privacy with each other. Communication skills are required in both relationships. The most significant difference is the helper's personal commitment, willingness to get involved, and use of the self to help others.

Because most nursing students have chosen the profession by being highly motivated to help others, they are apt to experience frustration about their powerlessness in numerous situations. Ultimately nurses need to recognize their limits, that their calling is not to cure everyone. They have to recognize that many problems have no solutions, that there may be clients who cannot find their way out of desperate situations and the nurse cannot either. Instead of being overwhelmed, nurses need to keep their distance and realize that every client has inherent strengths and that the nurse's task consists of letting the client rediscover those strengths and showing him or her how to use them.

The process used to achieve this is *empathy*. Certain writers hold that empathy is synonymous with active listening (Sorensen 1979:33–34), but in this book we view empathy as both the underlying emotional component and the active part of the listening process. The two aspects work together in the helping process. Empathy may exist without being expressed, but if a person is to be helped, the nurse should use active listening including empathy in order to communicate that the helper respects the client and is concerned. Attempts to help without communicating empathy are often misunderstood or resented by the person in need. A gift of money or material goods not accompanied by empathy, for instance, puts the client in the position of being needy or somehow inferior. People need dignity; pity does not provide it. Empathy is understanding the other person's situation, perceiving the nature of the other person's experience, and feeling respect for him or her as a person. At the same time, separate identities should be preserved (Rogers 1961:56); the nurse must protect himself or herself so as not to be affected by the client's pain.

Expressing empathy is using the self therapeutically. To do this, nurses need to be keenly aware of themselves, to compare themselves to the other person, to know what dynamics lead to happiness or sadness in themselves so that the nurses understand why certain dynamics make a client sad or happy. Such self-understanding is the principle on which self-help groups are based. People who are in the same boat understand and can be truly helpful to each other. The aim of empathy, however, is to understand clients who may be different from oneself. This process requires a mental effort. The nurse must consciously try to experience and feel as the client may feel.

No matter how different the helper is from the client, empathy consists in a search for commonalities. Helpers make a conscious effort to clarify the client's responses and to figure out how they would feel under the same circumstances. If the client does not express his or her feelings, helpers may tentatively describe what they would have felt. This serves two purposes. First, clients realize that they really matter to the helper and that the helper works hard to understand them. This is especially important, since people with emotional problems do feel misunderstood by their friends and the world. Second, it serves as a means to help clients learn about themselves. Often people who need help do not clearly perceive their own feelings; and by the helper's confronting them with what they may be feeling, they suddenly realize that they actually do feel angry or guilty.

Example:

HELPER: Tell me about the party last night.

CLIENT: I came in and nobody looked at me. I got myself a drink and stood there. A few people said "Hi," but they all had formed little groups and were busy talking.

HELPER: This made you feel lonely and out of place?

CLIENT: Yes. I felt that I was different and had nothing to say anyway.

HELPER: This sounds angry. You must have expected people to give you a warm welcome and then felt really disappointed.

CLIENT: I guess you're right. I always do that; I expect people to be nice to me. But of course they don't know me and therefore don't really care about me.

In this example, the simple situation told by the client and interpreted by the helper leads the client to an insight. He is about to realize that he cannot expect people to respond to him without disclosing himself to them in one way or another. While the client was talking, the helper had interpreted the client's problem. She probably remembered situations where she felt similarly or observed how she or other people handle such situations. She then draws from her own experiences.

Good helpers need to learn from everyday life, observe themselves and others, see relationships and orderly patterns, and be aware of interactions, needs, and feelings. Wisdom is the direct result of self-observation and self-awareness; textbooks cannot provide such knowledge. Helpers who have a good grasp on their own lives and know how to cope, either through their own experiences or observations of other people, will be able to pass some of their wisdom on to others through empathy and the helping process.

THE TEACHING PROCESS

The teaching process is part of the helping process. All concepts and principles discussed in this chapter should therefore be applied in the teaching process as well. Communication principles should be used to ensure clarity of the messages and understanding of the material taught. Empathy should be drawn on to provide congruence between emotions and the rational thinking process.

The teaching process has two components, teaching and learning. In a helping relationship, the helper does most of the teaching and the client does most of the learning. However, this is not exclusively so. The process is one of mutual participation, during which the client participates by giving feedback and providing input into the teaching process. The learning occurs not only by the teacher presenting the material and the client absorbing it, but by their mutually sharing the information and applying it to the client's life. The client's feedback helps the teacher to see the material taught from a different perspective. Talking with the client about the material lets the teacher recognize new points of view and new principles not previously thought of.

Certain conditions need to be present in order for the teaching-learning process to be effective.

1. The environment needs to be conducive to learning:
   - Cut out distracting noises such as those from TVs, stereos, and machines.
   - Provide comfort in lighting, temperature, chairs, and so on.
2. The client needs to be ready to learn:
   - Check his or her motivation.
   - Assess the client's ability to understand material.

3. The teacher needs to be skilled in the teaching process:
    - Use teaching techniques, AV material, practical demonstration.
    - Use empathy.
    - Include all family members, according to their level of understanding.
    - Use communication techniques.
    - Relate the material taught to the client's individual situation.

The environment cannot always be manipulated as the nurse might wish. Often the nurse enters situations that are in no way conducive to teaching. Such situations should be carefully assessed. Does the client have the power to change the situation? If yes, did he or she set up the situation in order to test the nurse? Under all circumstances the family should be told that the conditions are not good for the purpose of learning. If community nurses recognize that changes can be made with little effort, they should refuse to do the teaching, instruct the client to make these changes, and set up a date for a future teaching session.

Examples

A nurse wanted to teach a family a sensible diabetic regime for their 12-year-old daughter. When he entered, he did not find the daughter at home; she had been invited to a friend's house. The husband was drinking beer with a buddy from work, and the two were telling each other jokes. They asked the nurse if he knew some jokes. The mother was watching TV, the volume turned up so that she could still hear over the men's laughter.

The nurse explained that he could not do the teaching now, since the situation was distracting everyone and he needed the daughter present in order to present material about her diet. The family seemed to understand this. He then continued: "Since the diet is extremely important for your daughter's future health, all family members need to participate in changes and help her with them. Could I set up another appointment to see the two of you and your daughter at a time when you have no work to do or social obligations?"

Such assertiveness showed the family that nursing care was valuable and needed to be taken seriously. It also showed them that the nurse valued his own skills and time, and his action earned him status. At the same time, he had been careful not to hurt their feelings by letting his voice reflect anger or resort to any punitive statement. The response he wanted from them was not guilt but cooperation.

Other situations need to be accepted with more leniency. A young mother with four children who cannot afford a babysitter may have to be taught in her home in spite of frequent interruptions. However, if the nurse tells the mother that the condition is not ideal and that the teaching process suffers, she may be willing to tell her friends not to call during nursing visits or to set up the appointment at a time when the two little children are taking a nap.

At times, nurses do not encounter motivation to learn among clients and they must decide either to leave the family alone or to try to get them motivated. Nurses need to recognize that every family has the right to be left alone and to refuse nursing care. This right should be granted unless the reason for visiting this family is essential for their health and well-being. However, before nurses give up, the motive for refusing the visit should be carefully examined. The lack of motivation could stem from a blunder in communication, offensive behavior, or lack of empathy on the part of the nurse. It could also be a way of testing whether the nurse really cares. In some instances, the family may have a strong dislike of the nurse that is based on racial prejudice, past experiences with the health care system, or other emotional factors. The attempt at teaching should only be given up after the nurse has put genuine empathy to work and if the client has rejected this attempt. Even then, the attempt should be continued (as in the example of Sheila in Chapter 7) if the client is in a needy situation.

Fostering readiness to learn is difficult in cases where the client is noncompliant. The example of Robert Fox (Chapters 1 and 2) suggests the importance of assessing the client's true needs: only after these emotional needs were met would Robert listen to the nurse's teaching.

The points to remember in the process of motivating the client are:

- Use empathy, communicating a caring attitude.
- Listen carefully to how the client perceives the problem.
- Understand the client's point of view.
- Assess what emotional factors play into the client's refusing to change.
- Assess what needs the client meets with his or her behavior.
- Find ways to meet these needs in other ways.
- Get the client actively involved in finding solutions to meet these needs.

When the client's needs are satisfactorily taken care of, he or she will be ready to work on changes and will listen when the nurse explains the problem and necessary changes.

Example

The following demonstrates one of the hardest situations that can be encountered by a nurse.

Tracy Allen is in second grade, but she has problems in school because, although her intelligence seems satisfactory, when she has to learn something new she tries only once. If she does not succeed, she gets angry and frustrated and starts crying. Her attention span is quite short, and several times a day her teacher finds her sitting and just staring into space. In addition, Tracy is a loner and has difficulties being part of a group. She seems rather suspicious and has not formed close relationships with classmates or the teacher. She is short-tempered with other children and overreacts if someone criticizes her.

The school has ordered psychological testing for Tracy and and asked the community nurse to visit the parents for an assessment of the family situation. When the nurse arrives, the first question Mrs. Allen asks is, "Who sent you?" Told that the school did, she became very cold, and said, "I've had nothing but trouble with this school. Tracy hates the teacher and the school and that's why she has problems. I tried to talk to the teacher, but she wouldn't listen. Tracy needs a special teacher. She has a learning disability, but this school has not figured that out yet."

Seeing that the worst thing she could do would be to defend the school or the teacher, the nurse realizes Mrs. Allen is frustrated, feels misunderstood, and needs someone to listen to her. In addition, the nurse suspects Mrs. Allen needs to blame something for the trouble, such as the school's denial of a learning disability, and wonders if an emotional problem was threatening to her. She realized the mother's hostility toward her was not personal.

"I have watched Tracy today in class," she says. "She is a lovely girl and she is able to do some good work in school. I saw her attempt her spelling test, but after two words she threw the paper on the floor and cried. I went over to comfort her; her body was shaking, she was so upset. I'm concerned about Tracy; I think she deserves to be a happy girl. I came to see you in hopes that together we could find some way to help her."

Note that nurse has made sure not to throw in any judgments with regard to Tracy's problem. She has figured that most parents want their child to be happy and if she can offer help, perhaps Mrs. Allen will think it worth a try.

The statement turns out not to be enough, however, for Mrs. Allen responds by getting very angry; she tells the nurse that Tracy's problems are all due to the school and that she has done everything she could. The nurse sees that Mrs. Allen's response actually is quite positive: she expressed her emotions, which she would not have done if she had not felt trust.

When Mrs. Allen stops, she says, "You are very angry, and I can see a few reasons for making you feel that way. I can imagine that this trouble with Tracy and the school must take a lot out of you. I bet you had some troubles too even before Tracy went to this school. You're a very busy mother, with two other children and working, too. How do you manage all the work? It must be hard."

Mrs. Allen's anger has told the nurse that the real problem with Tracy is probably connected to Mrs. Allen's needs. The mother appears to be a needy person who feels desperate and misunderstood, and who projects her anger toward the school because the school people she has worked with in the past seemed to have consciously or unconsciously blamed her for Tracy's problems. The nurse has therefore decided to get to know Mrs. Allen and show concern for her problems rather than focusing on Tracy.

Mrs. Allen tells the nurse some things she is doing, about work and the other children. She has, however, carefully avoided any mention of Mr. Allen. Noting this, the nurse then asks Mrs. Allen whether she may come back and talk more some other time. She had waited until she had the feeling that Mrs. Allen started to enjoy sharing with her and that a beginning trust relationship was forming. She recognizes that Mrs. Allen needs to stop denying that her own life and her problems have a direct relationship with Tracy's problems. In order to get her to that point, however, the nurse needs to tend to Mrs. Allen's problems through empathy. Unless the nurse is able to express to her that her feelings and reactions are legitimate, Mrs. Allen will not admit to what has gone on within the family.

On every visit the nurse learns a little more. Eventually she sees that Mrs. Allen seems to be looking forward to the visits and is eager to tell about her troubles with her husband. Mr. Allen, it develops, is unemployed and has made the family suffer, especially Tracy, who cannot seem to do anything right for him. When Mrs. Allen cries about her marital relationship and Tracy's fear of her father, it is clear that she realizes Tracy's problems have been their problems and vice versa.

The nurse proposes play therapy sessions with Tracy in which Mrs. Allen can watch without participating and afterwards they can discuss what went on. During the activity Tracy expresses hatred and makes the father puppet drop dead. The nurse stresses that it is important for Tracy to get her anger out and that Tracy and her parents need to learn to communicate. Mrs. Allen admits that she has contributed to the problems in her own way, by encouraging Tracy's hatred of her father and fostering her dependency. Eventually, Mr. Allen is included in the discussions; after they both see their problems clearer, they agree to a family therapy referral.

The teaching in this example consists of making Tracy's parents aware of the interaction dynamics and their influence on the behavior of the family members. The nurse was acutely aware of the family's values as well as her own, a skill which has promoted empathy and understanding. The teaching process is inseparably mixed with active listening and the parents' coming up with conclusions without realizing that the nurse has actually led them that way. Teaching of general principles in mental health is interspersed. The nurse brings up these principles when they are needed to explain a phenomenon and they are applied to the individual problems.

This last point is the reason why nursing teaching often is more effective than teaching through mass media, for, correctly done, it brings about actual change. Most people know at least something about a healthy diet or prevention of cardiac disease through television, newspapers, pamphlets, and so on, but the knowledge brings about little change. Media teaching needs endless reinforcement before somebody actually stops smoking, for example, and even then the decision is usually influenced by some other person, someone who has stopped and now feels better or someone who really cares. The same is true for the alcoholic who makes the decision to stop drinking. The media is excellent for teaching the facts, but for the client's denial to be broken, empathy is needed; someone needs to care. For a client to change, the change has to make a difference in someone else's life as well as in his or her own. Most therapy programs today recognize this and involve the family and friends in the treatment process.

Nurses need to use their own empathy as well as the family members' for each other, if change is to succeed. This is why teaching within a family or within a group is more effective than from person to person.

The teaching process consequently consists of two aspects:

- Teaching the facts
- Interpretation and application

Whether facts need to be taught has to be assessed beforehand. Often clients know the facts from other sources, but it is wrong to assume that they do. Many times after a doctor has told clients about their disease they really do not know. Many factors could have prevented them from understanding: nervousness, preoccupation, inability to understand the medical terms, and so on. As stressed in Chapter 4, an assessment needs to be made to determine how much clients actually know. The nurse should then use audiovisual material, pamphlets, models, charts. Children should learn by doing, and the nurse should let them fill up their own syringe, drive dolls to the hospital in a toy ambulance, and she should find other new and different ways of teaching and demonstrating.

Nurses also need to keep in mind the client's attention span. The amount of material to be covered in one session should be reasonable. At least half of the time period should be used for the client to give feedback and ask questions. During a one-hour session it seems reasonable to use a few minutes for socialization, then present some 20 minutes worth of material, and spend the rest of the time with interpretation, application, and clarification. While teaching, the nurse needs to observe clients carefully. Their nonverbal behavior will give clues as to whether they are paying attention to what is said, are interested, and are ready to hear more. Eyes wandering, yawning, wiggling in the chair, and the like may tell the nurse that clients' attention span is used up. Getting up frequently, constantly paying attention to a child, changing the subject may tell the nurse that clients would rather talk about something else. Many of these reactions can be prevented by asking clients their opinion, letting them repeat to the nurse what they heard, and asking what they already know about the subject. The presentation of the material is more lively and more interesting if it is broken up, which means that a small section of the material should be presented, interpreted, and applied before the next section is presented.

Example:

> NURSE: Do you know what blood pressure actually is?
>
> CLIENT: It has something to do with the heartbeat. The blood gets pumped around.
>
> NURSE: Yes, and the pressure of the blood that gets pumped around is measured. The blood is in the arteries and pushes against their walls. You have these arteries in your arm and all through your body. *(Points to the client's arm.)* Arteries are in a way like pipes. If you have a thick pipe you get water through easily. But if you want to get the same amount of water through a thin pipe, what happens?

CLIENT: You need a lot of pressure.

NURSE: Yes, and it splashes out at the other end, doesn't it? *(Both laugh.)* Arteries can be either thick or thin. They have muscles that contract and relax their walls. When they are contracted, your blood pressure goes up; when they are relaxed, the pressure goes down.

CLIENT: What makes them contract or relax?

NURSE: If they are not stimulated, they are relaxed. Several things make them contract. The most common one is stress. Stress causes the body to secrete adrenalin, a hormone. Adrenalin works on the small arteries, the arterioles, and contracts them. Do you know what adrenalin is good for?

CLIENT: I've heard you have a lot of it when you're angry.

NURSE: Yes. The hormone is part of a response we have when we get excited, angry, scared, or nervous from stress. It's the same in animals. It prepares them to either fight or run away. The arterioles are clamped down to get more blood to the organs like the heart and the lungs where it's needed when the animal runs or fights. We have the same reaction even if we don't run or fight.

The teaching process is a mutual process during which the client actively participates. The nurse teaches only what the client is ready to hear and the material is taught in a way that the client understands, considering his or her mental ability, concentration, and motivation. Unfortunately, this most important principle is the one that most often gets violated. Some community nurses perceive their role as being a teacher who knows all and the client as the inactive pupil. Nurses who teach in this fashion are lecturing, preaching to the client. They find themselves giving advice the client has not asked for and solving problems the client has not defined. Such nurses are not well liked since they neglect to meet the client's needs. Though the clients may be courteous enough to listen, they are still most likely not to apply the teaching to their daily routines. Such practice is especially unacceptable if the nurse spends the session threatening them with what will happen if they do not change. Clients resent being parented by the nurse and they resent being made to feel that they have misbehaved. Teaching without understanding of the client's problem and without empathy does more damage than good.

SUMMARY

The building blocks for an effective working relationship are communication, the helping relationship, and the teaching-learning process. All three are closely intertwined, none being possible without the other two. Communication is the most important tool and consists not only of verbal exchange but skills in listening and perceiving the client's needs and keen observation of nonverbal cues coupled with the nurse's awareness of his or her own feelings and values. The helping relationship is born of effective communication and empathy for the client. Feelings for the client and understanding of cultural, racial, and other differences are basic also to the teaching-learning process that leads to actual change. Many techniques can be used for teaching, but the most important facets are involving the client in the process, applying information to the client's individual situation, and attending to the client's emotional needs before or while going through the teaching process.

REFERENCES

Berne E: *Transactional Analysis in Psychotherapy.* New York, Grove Press, 1961.
Powell JJ: *Why Am I Afraid to Tell You Who I Am?* Chicago, Peacock Books, Argus Communication, 1969.
Rogers C: *On Becoming a Person.* Boston, Houghton Mifflin, 1961.
Sorensen KC, Luckmann J: *Basic Nursing: A Psychophysiologic Approach.* Philadelphia, Saunders, 1979.
Sullivan HS: *The Interpersonal Theory of Psychiatry.* New York, Norton, 1953.

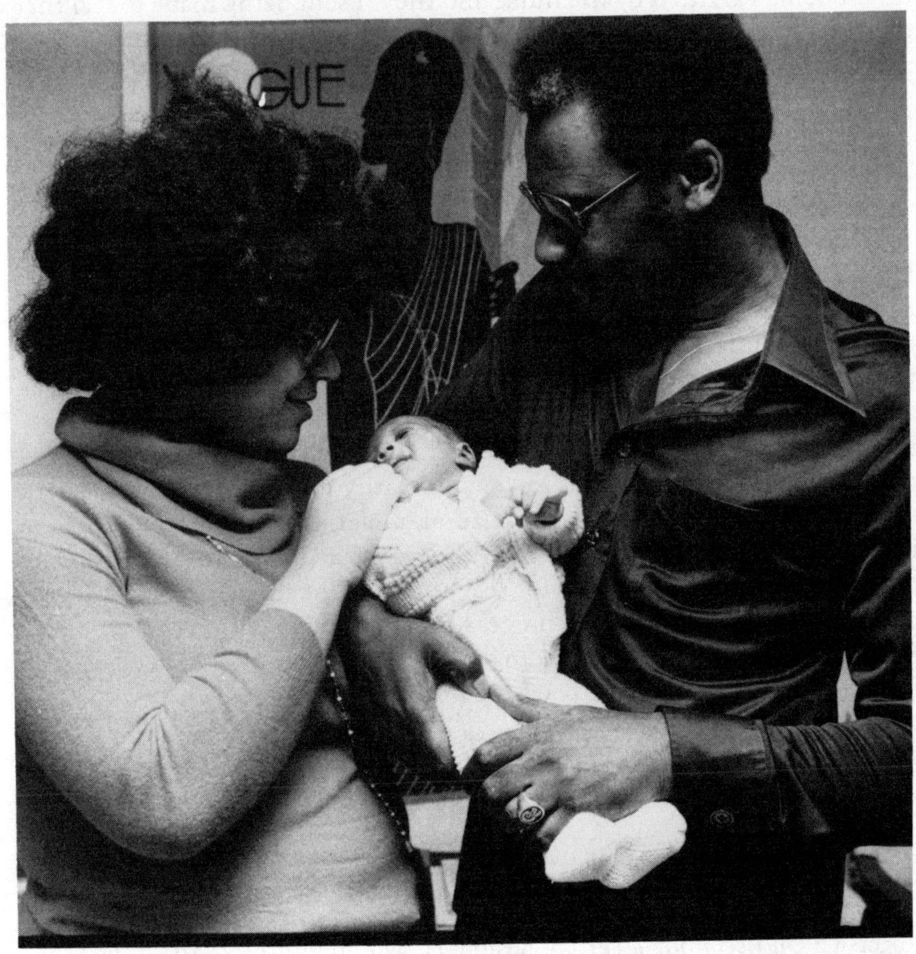

TYRON HALL/STOCK, BOSTON

IV

The Family

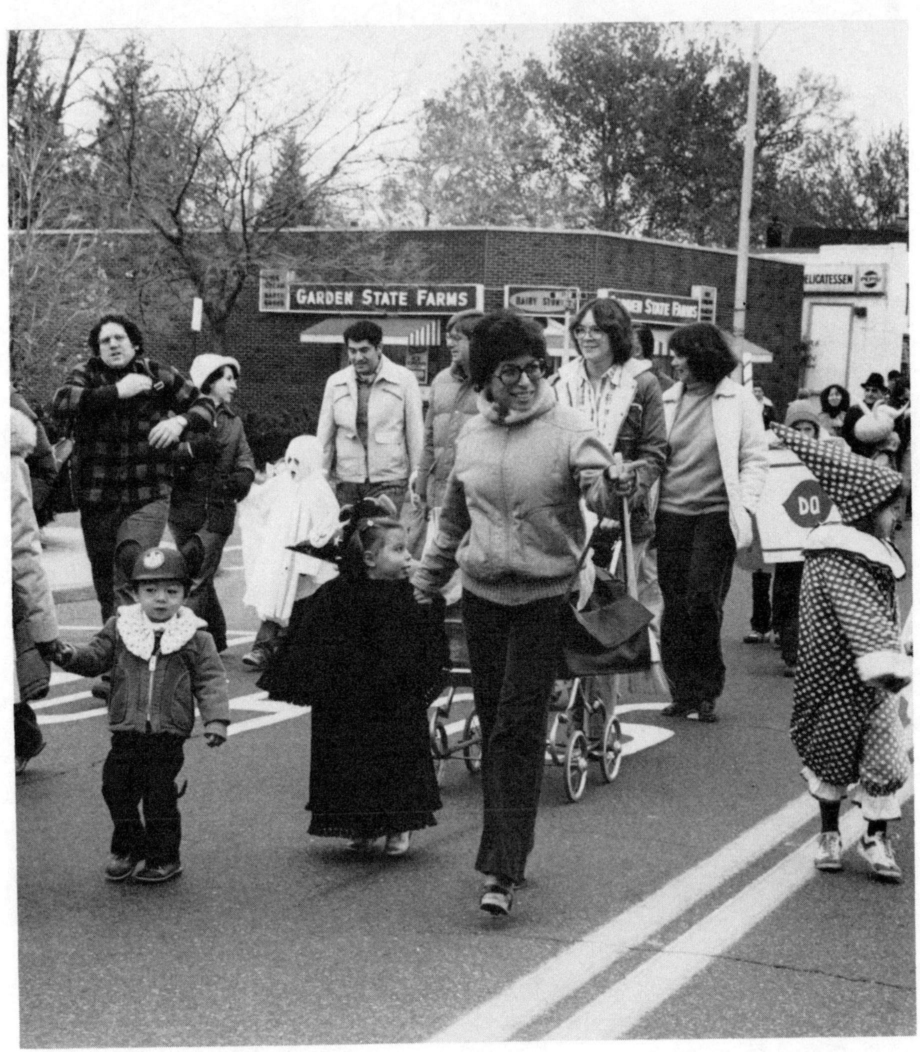

SYBIL SHELTON/PETER ARNOLD, INC.

10

Community-Family Relationships and the Individual

UNDERSTANDING THE COMMUNITY SYSTEM

The purpose of this chapter is to increase the community nurse's understanding of the forces that shape an individual. The unit within which a great part of this shaping takes place is the family. The family is not an independent system, however; it exists within the context of the community. This means that the individual is not only a product of the family but also of the community. There is an interrelationship between the three which the community nurse needs to understand. Only if the nurse understands how the three components work together can he or she make changes and understand why some people have fewer or greater options for change.

It is easiest to think of the community in Gottschalk's terms. (Gottschalk, 1975: Chap. 3) He sees the community organized in three levels, or circles, with the family at the center. The family level is surrounded by the community level, which is a network of social systems that serve basic human needs such as production, reproduction, consumption, recreation, and education. These social systems, which are the ones a family has contact with, are either loosely organized communal organizations, such as the neighborhood, a network of friends, or the extended family, or they are highly structured formal organizations, such as the place of work, the church, or the school. The third level, which encircles the other two, consists of external forces shaping people's lives. For instance, in times past, a farmer's family was fairly independent and self-sufficient, and outside happenings in the rest of the world did not concern them much unless the sons had to go off to war. Today everyone's life has become dependent in one way or another on the government, and the government in turn is often shaped by political happenings in other countries such as oil crises. Because of the thousands of social programs that affect great numbers of people, simple government decisions may change many lives, as was the case in extensive urban development in the 1970s, which caused many to lose their homes, neighborhoods, support systems, and even their identity—changes the extent of which lawmakers could not have realized. By getting involved in politics, community nurses can understand how all people—their clients as well as themselves—are affected by such happenings in the community and the world.

ECONOMIC FACTORS SHAPING THE INDIVIDUAL

That the physical environment shapes the individual can be seen in other countries, in which one becomes aware of the close association of people's environment and their lifestyles and as a result their social identity. In the United States, much has been written about the culture of the poor, which is adaptive and helps people living in unfavorable conditions to survive; however, this culture does not provide a child with optimal self-esteem and ego-integrity. Children use their family environments to build their identity; and it does not take slum children long to find out they are deprived. Even if they enjoy love and support from their families and security through a close-knit kin system, as they grow older their self-esteem is likely to suffer owing to lack of status. In school they have to identify with different standards and values and mix with children they have difficulties measuring up to intellectually. They see the discrepancies on television; if bused to another school, they perceive the status differences between themselves and their classmates even more vividly.

Benninger (1978: 382-388) points out the variables the optimal environment of any family should include:

- *Accessibility*—social and economic channels that give the individual the opportunity for self-realization.
- *Security*—the right to inhabit a dwelling place; and a chance for good health, employment, and a support system of family and friends.

- *Independence*—control over one's environment, which includes self-help and availability of services.
- *Identity*—sense of belonging through peer-relations, occupation, religion.
- *Status*—influence, respect by others, and self-esteem.
- *Potential*—ability to act in the future and growth of value over time.

Most people fall short in one or more of these factors. Freedom to choose an ideal living arrangement is limited by employment, education, economic, and personal factors.

By using Benninger's variables for the optimal environment, nurses can easily assess the extent of the discrepancy between the real and the ideal. The matrifocal family in the black ghetto, for example, is a product of poverty and deprivation and the social welfare system. The role of the male in the family is marginal, falling short on all of Benninger's variables. Accessibility is lacking owing to low education, no transportation to jobs, and poor job opportunities. Security is relative to employment, which is generally low paying and insecure. A person in the ghetto does not enjoy independence, as shown, for example, in the lack of availability of medical services; in most cities, such services are not in slum areas, transportation to them is difficult, the available clinics provide only impersonal treatment and superficial care despite long waits. Since the medical system does not meet their needs, slum residents do not use it often.

The black ghetto male's identity suffers if he compares himself with people outside the ghetto; his status is low, and his potential slim. Black women who are able to take advantage of the welfare system and receive AFDC for themselves and their children consider a husband a liability rather than an asset. (Crawford, T. 1971: 38) Since marriage means giving up public assistance, they have to be sure a husband's employment is sufficient support. The upshot is that females become independent and build ties with their children, whereas fathers do not have enough status to assume a leadership role. Women have another advantage in that their ability to have children is valued in their subculture. If they are not able to produce economically, having children assures them at least some status.

The economic factor not only decides behavior patterns in the ghetto, it permeates family and community life, also. It determines in what neighborhood people live, what social organizations they belong to, what schools they go to, what friends they have, whom they marry, and the circle of friends children associate with, who are important in shaping their identity. The puritan work ethic still persists, and so, to the male in the family, employment and money provide a sense of self-worth.

McLaughlin (1979) describes the several effects of unemployment. The first, she says, is financial: change in lifestyle, decline in living standards, crippling long-term financial commitments. A man may be reluctant to seek or take an inferior job, since it means accepting a lower standard of living. Children feel inferior to their peers since they can no longer afford luxuries. Such adjustments represent a grief process. Adult family members hit by unemployment show a high incidence of depression. Financial stress aggravates stresses from other sources. Even though they might have longed for leisure time, now they do not enjoy it. Stress is transmitted to family interactions. Unmet personal needs lead to tension, and living together may become unbearable.

SOCIETAL CHANGES INFLUENCING FAMILIES

With the rising divorce rate and the increasing number of one-person households, the high rate of unemployment, and the influence of the women's movement, many women are entering the work force. Women 16 years and older occupy an increasing percentage of the work force, up from 49.6 to 50% from 1970 to 1980. (US Census, 1970; US Census, 1980) About one-fifth of these working women have children between ages 6 and 17 and another sixth have children age 6 and younger. (US Census, 1980)

There seem to be two categories of mothers working—those who do so for economic reasons and those who consider work psychologically fulfilling. Traditionally, a mother's place was believed to be in the home. But housework is not highly valued in our society and does not provide status, and new trends influenced by the women's liberation movement give women a choice to venture out and find gratification outside the home. Adjusting to the world of work, however, depends on a woman's own values. For a woman working for strictly economic reasons, guilt feelings about not fulfilling her duties can lead to problems of ambivalence and inner conflicts. She may try to make up for "neglecting" her child, to become "Superwoman," performing two jobs and not giving herself time to relax. (Lancaster, 1975) Clearly, the responsibility of household and outside work places a great burden on the mother who does not want to delegate some of her chores to family members or helpers, and the resulting pressures are likely to cause anger, resentment, and even physical exhaustion.

Women who work for fulfillment rather than for purely economic reasons are likely to cope better and will have less guilt and feel freer to delegate their household duties. Unfortunately, the labor market is such that very few women (or men, for that matter) are actually in positions they enjoy. Today among full-time year-round workers, women's earnings still average 60% less than men's. Less than 25% of the discrepancy is accounted for by differences in education, experience, work commitment, or human factors. A significant part is due to job segregation by sex, resulting from the fact that women are concentrated in low-paying jobs. (Treiman and Hartmann, 1981) Women are moving into male-dominated professions, but progress is slow and is affected not only by lingering sexist attitudes of bosses and coworkers but also by women's own feelings of inadequacy and powerlessness.

A woman forced to work because of economic pressure and unable to find satisfaction on the job is unlikely to meet her needs, and this again may reflect on the child. Indeed, the impact may be stronger than the separation anxiety the child may suffer owing to the mother's absence, although research on the effects of working mothers on their children is conflicting. Rutter (1975), reviewing the literature, states that mother-infant bonding may be influenced by the mother's frequent absence, but the optimal length of time that a mother should spend with her infant cannot be determined. Infant-mother attachment seems to depend on how readily care providers can adapt their behavior to the specific requirements of the infant. Care providers are extremely important with regard to infant development, since the formation of children's attachment to the babysitter rather than the mother is a very real possibility and can lead to conflicts among the three. If there is a frequent change in sitters, says Rutter, and failure to form bonds, it may produce psychopathy in the child.

As the child gets older and is able to find support outside the nuclear family, the mother's absence seems to be less crucial, according to studies of school-aged children and adolescents during the '60s and '70s (Rutter, 1975). Sexual identification, especially of daughters, seems to be influenced away from the traditional roles as a result of identification with the mother. School performance seems to be good or better in these children. Negative effects on mental health does not find strong support. These studies, however, have been conducted with white middle-class women and did not include children whose mothers worked since infancy. In short, the field has not been researched enough to arrive at a clear understanding of the problem.

In addition, the roles of fathers have changed. Whereas fathers used to be the principal family breadwinners and authoritarians, today many share these duties with their wives and also those of child rearing. Indeed, child involvement often starts early, even before the birth of a child, with the father taking part in childbirth classes. Whether those changes have had large-scale effects on society's values and culture is not certain, but there seems to be a trend toward increased family involvement of young fathers.

These are just a few areas of the family and personal sphere which are affected by economics and other changes. In all these areas, however, causal relationships are not clear cut; many factors are involved, and many of them are not known. The dynamics are therefore hard to understand. In the case of working women, for example, economics is the determining factor for many but not for all. Some women go to work to fulfill personal needs—that is, to use their potential. These needs may be stimulated by changing social values brought on by the women's liberation movement but also by economics, educational possibilities, subsidized child care, and government scholarships. These factors themselves were brought about by public demand, which indicates that perhaps the social values were changed even earlier.

Today a nurse should look at family dynamics in terms of change. Change happens in all families, of course, and the ones that resist change seem to be under more stress than the ones that adapt to it. On the other hand, many families change without contemplating the consequences. Many women going back to work are shocked to find how difficult it is to cope with the secondary changes. They come to realize how dependent the total family network is on their functions within the family. They may discover behavior changes in the children as a result of the new routine—some perhaps advantageous, as in the children becoming more reliable and self-sufficient, but some problematic if the children's needs are no longer being met. The relationship of working mothers to young infants and their infants' later development is simply not known, and mothers who move to take jobs need to know that they are taking a risk. A nurse can make them aware of the infant's needs for mothering and help them select suitable child care arrangements.

Thus, change, whether coming from without or within, may touch numerous facets of family life, and one of the most important may be religion. Some families still maintain religious traditions, even though it no longer permeates every facet of life as it used to. For many people, the church is a place where people feel accepted and understood, a place to share problems and to derive strength from the belief that someone is watching over and helping carry the burden. Religion makes pain and hardship easier to accept. Those who do not have religion for backup and comfort, however, need to find other ways of coping. For many deeply religious nurses, it is difficult to abstain from offering their own ultimate solution to clients, and there is nothing wrong with this—if the clients ask for it. However, if the family has found other ways for coping or if they are in the process of looking for ways to cope, religion should be offered as only one alternative among others. Forced evangelism is just another way to push individual values on the client, and in many instances it meets resistance and destroys the nurse-client relationship. Moreover, religion may not be truly beneficial to the client because the often-rigid standards set by religious groups may damage individuals' self-esteem, rendering them guilt-ridden, insecure, and unstable. The nurse thus should assess how clients interpret their religious beliefs and evaluate the effect of such beliefs on the clients' life and coping abilities.

SOCIETAL EXPECTATION AS A SOURCE OF PROBLEMS

The expectations of our society put much pressure on families, especially those that do not have satisfactory support systems. For instance, society expects husbands and wives to have children whether or not they are emotionally ready to. Men are expected to fulfill their family's needs, do house repairs, work in the garden, and be models for the children when they are tired from work and need nothing more than rest and quiet. Women still encounter stigma if they work outside the home or find themselves confused and lonely as well as disappointed when they stay in the suburbs taking care of the children. Often they do not find the fulfillment in child rearing that society leads them to expect they should. (Satir 1967: 21, 22)

In addition, children often run up against expectations of parents and society that they have difficulties living up to. The school expects them to perform, parents may want them to excel in sports, peers expect them to fight back. Children who cannot live up to such expectations, who do not get rewarded for the qualities they have but keep hearing about their inadequacies, will eventually show emotional consequences. The education system seems to be structured for the intelligent, competitive student who earns rewards by performing well, but competitiveness does not work for children with low self-esteem. Children who live within dysfunctional family dynamics may feel insecure and troubled, preoccupied with meeting their needs rather than with learning, and every failure may contribute to their feelings of unworthiness. Peers are often extremely quick to pick up on such insecurity and their cruel teasing and tricks may further harm the children.

The factors described up to this point—economics, societal change, and societal pressure—all have a strong effect on family functioning, but there are other pressures as well—what Gottschalk (1975:19) calls forces from the external level. One of the most important is demographic change.

DEMOGRAPHIC CHANGES AND THEIR EFFECT ON FAMILIES

The total US population was 226.5 million in 1980. Though it slightly more than doubled in 25 years, the fertility rate has decreased from 1997 children in 1970 to 1301 per 1000 women of childbearing age in 1980 (US Census, 1970, 1980), to the point where it is below natural replacement of the population. The age profile is therefore changing. This trend is based on the spread of birth control as well as changes in attitude toward raising children. On a farm, children were an asset, but today in the city they constitute a liability in terms of money and effort. In addition, psycho-analysis has made people aware of the difficulties of parenting and the responsibilities involved in raising children. As a result, many people, since they have a choice, will have either few children or none at all. Economic stress and uncertainty influences this trend, as well as massive campaigns through the news media to cut down the birth rate.

Population distribution is also shifting. In 1950, there were 168 metropolitan areas, which represented 7% of the land area and 56% of the population of the United States. By 1975 there were 243 metropolitan areas, representing 14% of the land area and 73% of the population. During the 1970s, the total central city population declined to 43% of the metropolitan population and suburbia increased to 57%. Increase in the white population occurred mainly in the suburbs, while blacks there still represent only 5%. Fifty-six percent of the black population in the city live in poverty and represent about 75% of the total black population.

People migrating out of the city have a greater variety of jobs to choose from and have a higher income (Hersh, 1978: 56). This trend presents great problems for the metropolitan areas, which are running on tight budgets owing to lack of revenue. The causes of this trend are probably a combination of racism and the obsolescence of the cities, which were built for a different population. The question of moving out or not is mainly a financial one, and people left behind in the city may feel unhappy about not being able to achieve the better life outside their reach.

The effect of such influences is felt increasingly in today's families. In times past, most problems were dealt with by the extended family and by the church. Today the nuclear family finds less and less support, while stress increases. Since decisions are made elsewhere and lives are ruled by uncontrollable forces, there is a general mood of apathy settling over the population. Since people feel they make no difference with regard to the total community, they do not feel part of it. Instead they separate from common goals, feel alienated, and their main preoccupation is the fulfillment of their needs. Many people try to forget their conflicts through alcohol, drugs, sex, and various amusements.

Even though the family unit is vulnerable and in many cases in jeopardy, it is still the locus of the shaping of the next generation. Any nurse contemplating the effects of external change and stress will easily detect that such stress next affects the marital relationship of a couple and after that the children.

Satir (1967) points out that if a marital relationship is dysfunctional, parents often use the child to maintain their self-esteem. They need to feel that the child likes them. If the child disapproves of them, they are disappointed. Discipline thus becomes difficult. Often children find themselves caught between conflicting demands, anxious about being rejected by one parent for siding with the spouse. Parents often find it less threatening to use children as a vehicle through which hostility can be conveyed indirectly to the other partner.

Such children find that being loved is conditional. By loving one parent, they get disapproval from the other. They do not have security but instead live under constant fear of losing a parent. This fear is real in today's society. Divorce rates were estimated at 4.6 per 1000 people in 1974 and 5.2 in 1978. (Kalter, 1977; *Reader's Digest,* 1980) Since these figures only show the number of divorces in relation to total population, they do not reflect all the second and third marriages and all the pain and anguish that went with each previous divorce. Kalter states that of 400 children referred to an outpatient psychiatric clinic one third were from divorced families.

It seems likely that children of single parents are more vulnerable even if the divorce trauma is not counted. If single parents suffer social isolation owing to social stigmas (especially if a racial stigma is added), it may be detrimental to the child. Adjustment depends on meeting the psychological needs of parent and child. Economic aspects and community support are closely intertwined and related to the adjustment process.

Considering this incredibly complicated network of problems influencing and reinforcing each other and the extreme difficulties some families face in maintaining their homeostasis, one can easily recognize that the nurse willing to help them out of their chaos of confusion and powerlessness does not have an easy task. The first step toward effective intervention, however, is to think in terms of systems and factors that are interrelated and that influence the individuals. Then the nurse should attempt to conceptualize the family situation, including all known intervening variables, and to understand thoroughly their relationship. These factors should be kept in mind when reading Chapter 11, since they have a direct bearing on family interactions in that they influence the way in which family members attempt to meet their needs.

REFERENCES

Benninger CC: *Situations and Settings: A Search for an Optimal Development,* in Anthony EJ, Koupernik C (eds): *The Child in His Family.* New York, Wiley Interscience, 1978, vol 5, 375–388.

Dutton DB: Explaining the low use of health services by the poor: Costs, attitudes or delivery systems. *American Sociological Review* 43: 348–368, June 1978.

Gottschalk SS: *Communities and Alternatives: An Exploration of the Limits of Planning.* New York, Wiley, 1975.

Hersh SP: *Children and their families in the USA: Three profiles of change, with a commentary on stress, coping and relative vulnerabilities,* in Anthony EJ, Koupernik C (eds): *The Child in His Family.* New York, Wiley Interscience, 1978, vol 5, 55–69.

Howell M: Employed mothers and their families: Part 1. *Pediatrics* 52:256, August 1973.

Kalter N: Children of divorce in an outpatient psychiatric population. *American Journal of Orthopsychiatry* 47(1): 40–51.

Lancaster J: Coping mechanisms for the working mother. *American Journal of Nursing* 75: 1322–1323, August 1975.

McLaughlin B: When Daddy loses his job. *Nursing Mirror* 149(17): 25–27, October 18, 1979.

Reader's Digest: *1980 Almanac and Yearbook.* Pleasantville, NY, Reader's Digest, 1980.

Rutter M: *Maternal Deprivation Reassessed.* Harmondsworth, Middlesex, England, Penguin Books, 1975.

Safa HI: The matrifocal family in the black ghetto: Sign of pathology or pattern of survival?, in Crawford CO (ed): *Health and the Family: A Medical-Sociological Analysis.* New York, Macmillan, 1971.

Satir V: *Conjoint Family Therapy.* Palo Alto, Calif, Science and Behavior Books, 1967.

Schwartz EB: Psychological barriers to increased employment of women. *Issues in Industrial Society* 2: 69–73, November 1971.

Treiman DJ, Hartmann HI (eds): *Equal Pay for Jobs of Equal Value.* Washington, DC, National Academy, 1981.

US Department of Commerce, Bureau of the Census: *Female Family Heads,* Current Population no. 50, Washington, DC, US Government Printing Office, 1971.

US Department of Commerce, Bureau of the Census, *1980 Census of Population and Housing.* Washington, DC, 1980.

US Department of Commerce, Bureau of the Census, *1970 Census of Population and Housing.* Washington, DC, 1970.

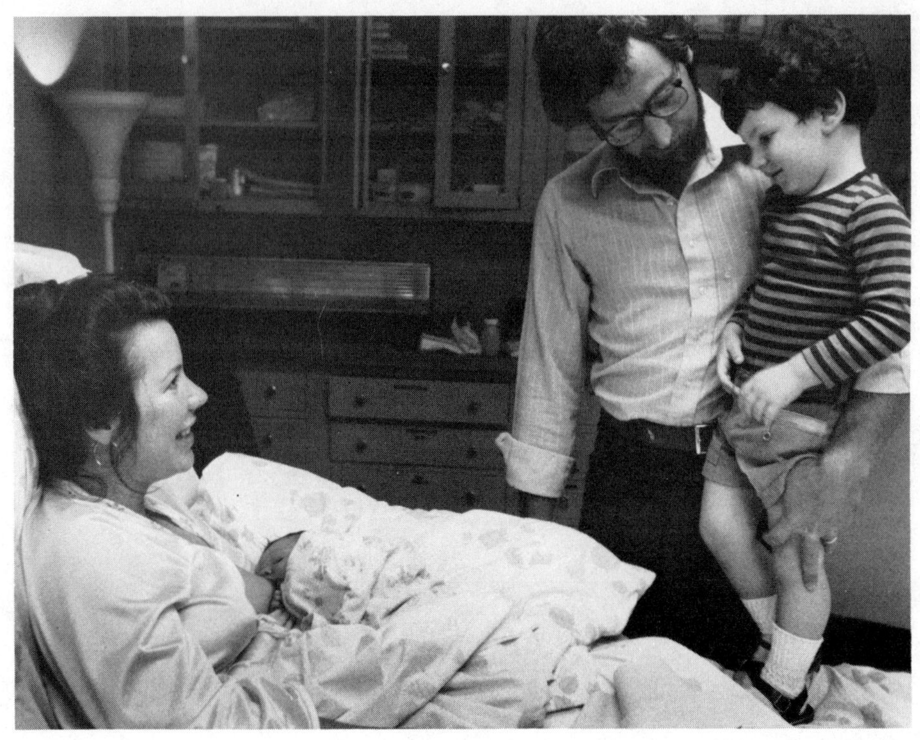

MARIETTE PATHY ALLEN/PETER ARNOLD, INC.

11

Patterns of Interaction

As previously pointed out, the family needs to be looked at as a unit in its own right. Research on schizophrenics who have been labeled delinquent members of their families has shown that the role of the delinquent seems to serve a purpose. Family members tend to resist and sabotage the individual treatment of the afflicted member; if that member gets better, other family members often get worse. (Satir:2) These findings clearly show the family cannot be evaluated objectively by looking at the members independently.

Probably the main reason why families have survived throughout the stresses of the twentieth century is that people's basic needs are met best within a well-functioning family. Loneliness is painful, and most human beings have a basic longing to be understood and to share their life experience with intimate friends. In an unstable, rapidly changing world, close ties with others become increasingly important. Throughout history, kinship ties have been most stable and most durable. Today many families are failing, and no longer withstand the stresses imposed on them that we discussed in Chapter 10. Many members of the younger generation do not have adequate role models or skills to make a relationship work. Many are troubled with underlying psychological problems that prevent sharing, intimacy, or giving to others. These problems are on the increase and can be verified by looking at the steadily increasing divorce rate.

In spite of failure, the family persists, probably owing to people's basic longing for harmonious family life. The majority of people who have failed in a marriage try again and again, even though their situation gets more and more complicated as children are combined from different marriages and shared with ex-partners.

Even though the vast majority of families are traditional—that is, they are headed by men—community nurses will find units of different structure. In 1980, 5.6 million white families and 2.3 million black families were headed by women; many couples live together without being formally married; a small percentage of people live in nontraditional household groups, loose friendship groups, homosexual unions; and 18 million people live alone. (US Census, 1980) Whatever the set-up, it represents an attempt by the people involved to meet some basic needs, and the community nurse's judgment about it should be based solely on how well these needs are being met.

THE FAMILY AS A FUNCTIONING UNIT

In trying to understand the family, a nurse needs to think of it in terms similar to those for the individual person. Just as people are similar in some ways and different in others, families are too. With this in mind, the nurse can evaluate how a family functions and how homeostasis is maintained. This understanding is essential for two reasons: First, it allows the nurse to look at problems and strengths objectively, since the family unit acts as a modifier by either intensifying or dampening the effect of internal and external influences. Second, it allows the nurse to intervene more effectively in using the family resources or in deciding on a referral if the family's problems are too great.

Walton-Spradley (1981:232) lists the most important similarities:

1. Every family is a small social system.
2. Every family has its own cultural values and rules.
3. Every family has structure.
4. Every family has certain basic functions.
5. Every family moves through stages in its "life cycle."

It should be added that:

6. In every family, members assume definite roles and communication patterns.

Differences between families have the same characteristics:

1. Every family handles boundaries, system input, throughput, and output in a unique way.

2.   Rules and culture are different for every family.

3.   Structure shows variation between families.

4.   Every family meets basic functions in a unique way (or fails to meet them).

5.   Families have reached different stages along their "life cycle."

6.   Roles and communication patterns are unique for every family.

As a system, the family is in continuous interchange with the environment (see Chapter 10). This is necessary because it depends on the environment for input such as goods, education, and friends. Families do not want to be totally ruled by the environment, however; they are concerned about preserving their individual characteristics, which provide the members with a sense of belonging and identity. The term "family homeostasis" (Jackson, 1957) describes the state every family strives for. Ideally, a family has the resources to ward off problems and conflicts in an efficient way and return to the dynamic equilibrium, homeostasis, which provides safety for the members and takes care of their emotional needs. In order to prevent input from the environment from overwhelming the coping mechanisms, the family uses boundaries to regulate input.

Family Boundaries

The regulation of boundaries is unique for every family, and the appearance of neighborhoods is a striking example of such differences. If you walk through a Latino district in a large city on a warm summer weekend, you will see people gathered outside, with women knitting or preparing food for cooking, children playing, men discussing sports or watching TV on someone's porch. There will probably be a lot of noise—radios blaring, motorcycles, children screeching and women disciplining them. A white, middle-class neighborhood, by contrast, may give a completely different impression: it may seem deserted. People will be away for the weekend, although dogs may bark from fenced-in yards and families may be glimpsed inside the house watching a ball game on television. The structure of neighborhoods tells the nurse about family boundaries. Homes separated from each other with hedges and fences may be less likely to foster a spirit of cohesion among the neighbors. A family in such a neighborhood may be reluctant to allow a nurse in and may be more suspicious than a family in a more open neighborhood, where children circulate through everyone's backyard and feel free to visit neighbors' homes. Such neighborhood characteristics and family boundaries may be related to external conditions. A high crime rate may make people more suspicious of strangers and keep to themselves; they may have big, vicious dogs. However, some neighborhoods react to crime the opposite way, by becoming cohesive neighborhood groups, watching out for each other.

These examples point out that boundaries may be determined by several factors, such as culture, external threat, personal experiences, history, and present-day experiences. They also show that all family characteristics are interdependent, so that rules depend on the way the family functions, roles depend on the family structure or culture, family functions depend on the stage in the life cycle, and so on.

Boundaries also determine what people a family will reach out to and what resources in the community it makes use of. This is particularly important for the nurse concerned about referrals. Solutions that may sound ideal at first need to be examined to see if they are compatible with family boundaries. A client with a colostomy, for example, who has spent his life predominantly within the family, sharing very little with the outside world, may be the wrong candidate to refer to an colostomy self-help group. He may, however, profit from discussing his problem with his wife and daughters, to be reassured that they still accept him as a valuable family member. The nurse should find out from the family who will lend help in case of other problems or what agency their friends use, since a positive attitude is important for effective care.

Rules, regulations, restrictions, and limits set by the family may be determined by values and culture. They too are related to how the family interacts within and with the environment. Some families are permissive, allowing cats and snakes, long hair and curls, early dating and early sexual relationships, whereas other families place firm restrictions on their members. They may need these restrictions to preserve their identity against a hostile environment. For instance, they may feel different and be proud of being different, but this attitude may create problems for their children, who would like to be part of the larger community and so have to live two different and uncomfortable roles. The larger the discrepancy between family standards and the standards of the community, the more likely that family experiences stress and loss of equilibrium.

Family Approach to Problems

Reiss and Oliveri (1980) have conducted interesting research examining families' adaptive capacities when experiencing stress. Based on their studies, they were able to categorize family responses according to three dimensions: configuration, coordination, closure. By *configuration* they mean the family concept of how the world is ordered by principles that can be discovered and mastered. Families exhibiting high configuration are able to tackle problems by adjusting the behavior changes imposed on them by the environment. Families with low configuration adhere to antiquated behavior patterns and rituals through which they experience security and which they are unwilling to change. Changes experienced by the society will be rejected by the latter family and will cause severe stress.

Coordination is the ability of a family to solve problems as a group. The concept is positively related to cohesion; however, it is more specific in its focus on adaptation to external pressure.

Closure is the measure of the time a family takes to make a decision based on evidence to support that decision. A family high on the closure dimension will get input from as many family members as possible and will try to accommodate their needs. A family low on the dimension will solve problems according to preconceptions, rituals, and values; solutions for them require no effort and decisions are reached quickly.

This conceptual framework may help the nurse to look at a family in terms of its functioning. However, extreme care should be taken not to judge a family as functional on the basis of these dimensions alone, as the following examples show.

Example 1: The Knox Family

The Knox family has an 18-year-old daughter. Annie is in her senior year in high school and is pregnant. This causes great stress in the family. An unwanted pregnancy is considered undesirable by the parents, who have been raised with strict religious principles. The family is angry at society for loose morals, and at Annie for betraying the family and destroying its good name.

At the same time, the Knox family is a closely knit group. They tend to stand as a united front when facing threats from the larger society. When Mr. Knox was laid off, for instance, Mrs. Knox did domestic work and the children had summer jobs, earning their own money for clothes. When a member is sick, he or she is well cared for by the family. However, when the family heard the news of Annie's pregnancy, the father reacted by saying, "You don't belong here any more! Our family doesn't support whores!"

The nurse can see that this family ranks low on "configuration," high on "coordination," and low on "closure." The family reaches conclusions quickly, since the members react to a predetermined set of values. They perceive changes happening to the family as a threat. Their values are inflexible, passed on over generations. They exclude other alternatives to their way of life. The parents expect their children to sacrifice some individuality for the sake of the family. The children are well trained and well liked by the teachers. They perform in school and are helpful around the house. Little transgressions are forgiven after a good spanking, and the older children have to do some work to make up for it.

If a crisis such as Annie's pregnancy occurs, the nurse has to evaluate carefully what solution might be practical for all. The father's attitude needs to be tested after the first shock has passed. He may be placed in a conflict between two different sets of values—those of responsibility and caring for one's children and those of unacceptability of sexual transgressions within the family. An opinionated individual like Mr. Knox, however, is not likely to be influenced by a community nurse in this struggle. All the nurse can do is to give him permission to express himself verbally and bring his thoughts out in the open, which will indicate not only to the nurse but his wife where he stands. Mrs. Knox's opinion in the struggle is as important as Mr. Knox's; however, the power of her opinion depends on the power and authority status she has within the family. If Mrs. Knox firmly supports Mr. Knox's opinion, the nurse needs to realize that the solution obviously does not consist of acceptance of the daughter and her continued presence within the family. That is, the family will cope by actually ostracizing the daughter. Depending upon the power of their values, they would feel little or no guilt about their action, and they would actually feel relieved after the daughter moved out. The nurse would then have to concentrate her efforts on helping the daughter settle independently and find a way of living on her own.

In today's society such a family is rare. Most families seem to yield to the pressure of change within the society, at least to some extent. The above example, however, shows that the Knox family is vital and functional as a unit. Their way of coping is likely to be unacceptable to the community nurse, since it victimizes the daughter, but by excluding the delinquent member the family eliminates the conflict, saves face and reputation, and functions as before (except for anger and hurt feelings toward the daughter, who "does not exist anymore").

Example 2: The Feldcamp Family

The problem of a daughter's pregnancy in the Feldcamp family had very different results. Mary's announcement was received coolly. "The way you've been running around with boys, we expected it!" Mr. Feldcamp said. "Now you have it, do what you want!" Though angry, because his values found his daughter's pregnancy unacceptable, Mr. Feldcamp was a reasonable man. After calming down, he suggested that the family should convene that evening and decide what to do about the problem. A heated discussion occurred. Mr. Feldcamp thought an abortion would be best, since Mary was still in school and had no way of supporting a child. Mary vehemently opposed it, since she wanted to keep the baby. She also had no desire to get married, since she hardly knew the baby's father. Mrs. Feldcamp was not sure of her position, but knew that she did not want to take care of the child, since she was working full time and the family needed her income. She would have favored an abortion if it had not been against her moral principles. The discussion did not lead to any logical conclusion. Mary defended her position. Mr. Feldcamp angrily told her it was her responsibility. Mrs. Feldcamp supported neither of them.

Mary stayed in the house; however, the family relationship deteriorated. Communication was at a minimum. Mary looked for support outside the family and was rather unhappy. When the baby was born, Mary took him home. At first she was happy and excited about the baby, but after a while she felt the loss of her freedom. The other family members were not willing to change their routines. If Mary asked them to help her, they got angry and told her that it was her duty. Having to stay home with the baby and not getting support from the family caused Mary to be depressed. With no way to finish her education or reach future goals, she started to resent the baby who interfered with her life.

The Feldcamp family generally scores rather high on configuration. They attempted to discuss the problem, but a solution was not possible. The intervening factor is their coordination, which is low. This family has traditionally functioned by allowing every member to pursue his or her own happiness without giving much consideration to the other members. For example, Mary had been running around with boys, but no one had set limits or even talked to her about possible consequences. Closure was delayed indefinitely. The problem created friction, angry feelings, and communication breakdown. Every time a family member looks at the baby, he or she is reminded that, because of him, the family is no longer what it used to be. Mrs. Feldcamp watches the baby occasionally, but does so grudgingly, resentful about losing her freedom. Mary feels hurt about not being understood, loved, and accepted. Thus, the family unit no longer meets its members' needs, and homeostasis cannot be restored until a solution is found to the problem.

This shows that the three criteria with which to evaluate a family's functioning when it is faced by problems do not tell the nurse how vital and strong a family is as a unit. Some families are very low on coordination and function quite well. At times nurses have difficulty finding anything members have in common, yet on closer look find that they all want to live their individual ways and they mutually respect this wish. This conceptual framework does not serve to evaluate the family but to understand its functioning as a system.

In a system, members are interdependent and connected by emotional ties. A change happening to one member will have a spreading effect and demands adjustment of all other members. Coordination is positively related to this aspect of the system. Whereas interdependency and coordination holds true for all families, its dimensions are different. Coordination is only one aspect of a broader characteristic, that of an emotional basis, a feeling that one is part of and responsible for the family, that one is concerned about all family members and shares their jobs and their problems. In summary, the nurse should learn to look at the family as a system and think in terms of systems. Knowing that all families have certain characteristics in common, the nurse needs to explore the unique features about those characteristics.

The concepts discussed thus far give the nurse a handle on understanding the family as it functions as a unit; however, they alone do not tell whether the family is functional or dysfunctional. The two areas most conclusive in pointing out problems or strengths are the ones listed in the family-assessment section: roles and physical interaction, and communication. Both areas are tools for meeting a family's functions and members' needs and for determining whether or not these functions and needs are met.

ROLES AND INTERACTION PATTERNS*

The basic functions of the family, as listed by Duvall (1977: 114–116), are the following:

- generating affection
- providing personal security and acceptance
- giving satisfaction and a sense of purpose
- guaranteeing social placement and socialization
- inculcating controls and a sense of what is right

*This section adapted from Table 7-3 (p 144) and headings for six "Emergent Family Functions" (pp 114–116) in *Marriage and Family Development*, ed 5, by Evelyn Millis Duvall. Copyright © 1957, 1962, 1967, 1971, 1977 by JB Lippincott Company. Reprinted by permission of Harper & Row, Publishers, Inc.

In order to meet these functions, the family members need to take on the responsibility of performing the actions necessary to achieve them. Traditionally, the responsibilities have been shared between mother and father within prescribed roles. In her role the mother provides most of the emotional support and affection, which is mainly invested in the time she spends with her children; maintains a home, which provides security and a place where socialization can occur in a growth-promoting atmosphere; and is sex partner to her husband and companion to him and the children. She also introduces limits and controls, disciplining the children in ways that maintain their self-esteem and rewarding them for positive behavior. The father's main role, traditionally, is that of provider, since economic well-being is, of course, important to the family's physical and emotional well-being. He also supports the mother and helps with showing affection for and disciplining the children, for whom he is a role model, and he teaches their roles in society.

The children, then, need to conform to the standards set for them by the father and mother. They learn to obey what the parents tell them is right and get sanctioned for doing wrong. A positive emotional climate, a general sense of being accepted, and unconditional love help them to accept the standards rather than feel coerced into conformity and rebelling against it. They see a purpose in the rules and regulations. They also are expected to respect their parents and, depending on their stage of development, to help the family in any way they can, and to learn new roles and drop old ones as they get older.

In nontraditional families, the needs of the members may stay the same, but the roles may shift. In a one-parent family, for example, the mother or father becomes responsible for roles that were previously shared by two people. These are great responsibilities. Many single parents are able to compensate by pulling into the family boundaries a network of friends to serve as role models to the children, to provide affection to all, to help socialize them, and so on. Problems arise, however, if the single parent tries to play all the roles and take on all responsibility, therefore neglecting to meet his or her own needs.

Whether a family is functional or not depends less on who fulfills what role than that *someone* fulfills the roles. If the mother works, for example, the rest of the family needs to adjust; the mother can no longer be expected to do all the household duties and give emotional support, keep track of all the children's behavior, discipline them for transgressions, and at the same time meet her own personal needs. Such a move, if handled effectively, needs a change in the husband's role, such as his taking part in household and everyday duties. The children also need to help and to look out for each other. In addition, the time allowed for each other needs to be structured with more care, and everyone needs to make an effort to maintain communication in spite of the heavy schedule.

Dysfunctional Interaction Patterns

Again, it is not important who fulfills the role as long as the role is handled efficiently. Often, however, this is not the case. If one partner becomes dysfunctional, as happens in substance-abuse cases, or leaves, as in divorce cases, roles are often assumed by children who are not emotionally fit to carry the responsibility. The so-called role reversal leads to a child's actually taking care of the parent by trying to provide emotional support (which the child is really not equipped to do) or physical support to the dysfunctional parent, as when a young boy fetches his father home from the bar and puts him to bed. Role reversal is typified by child abuse as well. Because the parent did not experience love during his or her own childhood, he or she expects the child to take on the role of a caring "parent"; then, when the child does not live up to these expectations, he or she gets beaten (Kempe and Helfer, 1972:4). Role reversal often happens in situations in which a family member is mentally ill or has psychiatric problems such as depression, dependency conflict, anger, or aggression.

Another sign of dysfunction is the development of manipulative roles within the family, as happens when family members, in striving to meet their personal needs, resort to game playing. Perls (1979:42) describes the positions of "topdog" and "underdog." The topdog in the family is the one who rules the household and threatens the members who do not conform with punishment or loss of love. The underdog strives for power in different ways, playing at being helpless. He or she always "tries" but does not succeed, and it is never his fault; however, he or she usually outsmarts the topdog. This kind of social game can be observed frequently in families. It is played between husband and wife, father and son, mother and daughter, or among siblings. Example:

HUSBAND: How did you blow all that money in one day! I told you, we're not rich. I just can't give you any money from now on. You don't know how to handle it. You're ruining us!

WIFE: But honey, I was out shopping with Mary and Shirley. What would they think if I told them that I couldn't afford those things? They would think we're too poor to associate with.

HUSBAND: Who cares! We wouldn't lose much. I can't put up with this any longer. You do this again and you won't see *my* face around here any more!

WIFE: I'm so sorry, honey. I've tried so hard not to spend money during these last weeks. And I didn't know your feelings would get so hurt because of this shopping trip. I would have stayed home if I'd known.

HUSBAND: OK, now, I don't want this to happen again.

WIFE: Yes, dear, I promise.

Interactions in families do not always occur in dyads. Many interaction patterns boil down to what is called the family triangle. In a functional triad, the marital partners feel confident in their relationship. Their relationship is something unique and one from which the child is excluded. The child responds with a natural fear of being left out. This fear can be alleviated by allowing the child to form his or her own relationship with the father as well as with the mother and by both parents being accepting of the mate's relationship with the child.

Virginia Satir (1967, Chapter 7) outlines what happens when the family triangle is dysfunctional. The marital relationship is unsatisfactory and the partners do not meet their needs but feel alienated. Since they are disappointed, they use the child to meet their needs. They ask the child to side with them. Incest relationships are started with these same dynamics: the other-sex parent, disappointed with the sexual relationship with his or her mate, seduces the child, and this evokes jealousy in the spouse and disapproval of the close relationship. Because the child needs both parents, he or she therefore tries to make up with the other parent.

Even without a sexual motive, a child caught between the parents' arguments will become the center of attention of both parents and will come to believe that he or she is essential to making the relationship work. The parents need the child to gain self-esteem, but the child does not get his or her own needs met. In severe cases the parents' relationship may become the child's main behavioral motivation. That is, the child will adopt whatever behavior serves the purpose of holding the parents together yet not let them be too close so that he or she will be let in too. The child may use extravagant behavior and become sick or emotionally disturbed. Family therapists find that the victim of the family triangle as a rule is very willing to give up this behavior as soon as the marital relationship no longer puts him or her in the double-bind position.

Transactional analysis explains this same phenomenon with the "drama triangle" or "Karpman triangle" (Karpman, 1968), as shown in Figure 11-1. In this figure, P is the persecutor, R is the rescuer, and V is the victim. This action at times occurs during normal circumstances. For instance, a legitimate role for a persecutor would be to discipline a child for naughty behavior. The victim can legitimately be a child who has hurt his or her knee, or a father who has lost a job in spite of good efforts. The rescuer is the person who helps the hurt child with a Band-Aid or who helps the father with understanding and empathy.

However, as in the family triangle, when these roles become a repeated pattern in which the interactions circulate around the triangle, the dynamics become a game of manipulation. Consider the following example, in which Jimmy has hit his brother Bobby on the head:

FATHER: (PERSECUTOR)	You naughty boy! You always have to start fights! Get up to your room!
JIMMY: (VICTIM)	Waahhh!
MOTHER: (RESCUER)	What's going on? *(She hugs Jimmy.)*
JIMMY: (VICTIM)	Bobby was mean to me and so I hit him. Dad wants to send me upstairs—it's not fair!
MOTHER: (PERSECUTOR)	*(To Father)* You can't do this to him. Normal boys fight. Why do you get so upset? Just leave them alone, will you.
FATHER: (VICTIM)	I was only trying to do what's right. *(He angrily leaves the room.)*
JIMMY: (RESCUER)	Dad, don't be mad. I'm sorry I hit Bobby.

The situation here is synonymous with the family triangle. The marriage relationship is not stable. Jimmy manipulates the parents. He plays

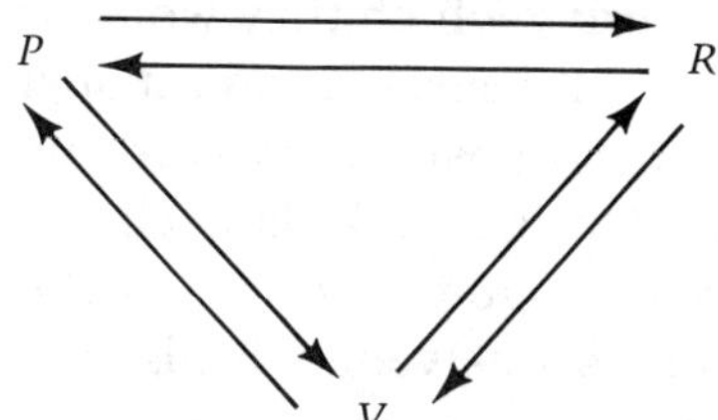

FIGURE 11-1.   The drama triangle.

them off one against the other. Often the initial provocative action has the purpose of setting up the game: Jimmy wants to be let in. He needs attention—and he gets it by hitting his brother. The father then gets angry. So far, the interactions are functional. The dysfunctional pattern shows in the mother's response. In a healthy family interaction pattern, the mother would not side with the son and contradict her husband. When this happens repeatedly, it usually means the mother has herself been a victim all along and is brought on by the mother's desire to get even. When the mother sides with Jimmy and the father gets angry, Jimmy realizes what he has done. Fearing that he might lose one parent, he attempts to reverse the pattern by getting Dad to love him again.

Children learn early to manipulate parents. As young as age two they run to the father after being scolded by mother. Parents need to agree on discipline policies and support each other in reinforcing them. The child in a healthy family does not have many chances to manipulate. Rules are set and understood by the whole family. Even older siblings support the rules set by the parents and they mutually control each other's behavior.

One of the most noticeable signs in young dysfunctional families is inconsistency in discipline. Inconsistent parents are those who often get tired of telling a toddler not to do certain things and let the child get by with something he or she got punished for the day before. The child, who is exploring his or her limits, finds that these limits are not set firmly and gets confused. He or she cannot understand why the mother reacts differently one day than she does on another, or why she allows children to turn the knobs on the TV sometimes and at other times slaps them for it. Insecurity leads the child to test the parent for reactions to certain types of behavior in order to try to predict parental behavior and feel more secure. If playing parents off against each other is the only way the child can alleviate fears of being ignored, he or she will resort to the necessary behavior to do so.

The problem is particularly severe with parents who are emotionally labile, such as depressed parents or substance abusers. Bothered by mood swings, they have days during which they would rather not have the child around. Such parents are self-centered and get angry about being bothered by toddlers. They are in no position to meet the toddlers' needs or to discipline them firmly. During such days children are likely to act up because they need attention and need to feel they are important to the parents. The parents' unresponsiveness leads them to all kinds of behavior, since often children prefer an angry parent to one who pays no attention at all.

Diagnosing Family Dysfunction

If a nurse discovers that a young mother is inconsistent in disciplining her child or not strict enough in consistently enforcing limits, it may be tempting to think that all the mother needs is to be told to enforce discipline, that she need only be told what will happen to the child if she does not change. Unfortunately, in most cases this approach is inadequate. The mother's behavior needs to be viewed in family system terms. The roots of this mother's behavior could be of a different nature. Perhaps she has an emotional problem or feels depressed and tired and not up to giving good mothering. Perhaps she is plagued by stress from the outside or from the marital relationship. Perhaps she lacks the self-confidence to enforce rules with the child. Before the actual change in disciplining methods can be tackled, the nurse needs to make a thorough assessment and with the help of the mother determine what the roots of the problem are and what changes need to be made within the underlying dynamic structure.

While methods of disciplining are often indicators of how a family functions, the nurse has to be careful about making premature judgments. Discipline is strongly influenced by culture. Before a family can be labeled dysfunctional, the nurse needs to determine the norm within the ethnic group the family belongs to; some cultures discipline children physically, others use different methods. In addition, the nurse should realize that the line between spanking and child abuse is a fine one. Even a well-adjusted parent will get some release of tension by spanking his child, but child abusers punish to satisfy their own needs. The parents' feelings need to be explored as well. Do they think they are handling their children well and are able to control them? The chance that they are abusing children is much greater if they feel that children are unusually naughty and uncooperative and they cannot seem to get them to mind. The standards parents put on their children need to be looked at. Are they within reasonable limits for the particular age range or do the parents expect too much of their children? Do the children have to perform to satisfy the parents' egos?

Discipline is not the only indicator for family functioning. Other aspects of parent-child interaction may be equally revealing. Parent-child interactions should be judged according to the extent to which they meet the child's needs and in turn the extent to which the parents' needs are met through the child.

Hollingshead (1941:55−56) lists a child's needs in his well-known theories of socialization, which are related to Maslow's needs but geared to the child:

1. Bodily needs: The infant is forced into the presence of human beings and he or she will become like them.

2. Craving for security: The child finds satisfaction if he or she is loved and unhappiness if affection is denied. The child is driven by a need for social prestige and acceptance and does those actions that gain approval. Disapproval by peers is a serious blow; this need causes the child to conform and form morality.

3. Need for activity and new experiences.

Whether the child's bodily needs are being met is relatively easy to observe. The nurse should assess whether the child is dressed adequately for the climate and temperature, is reasonably clean, is active and outgoing. Physical appearance may indicate nutritional status: a pale child with observable tooth decay may have a diet deficient in iron and high in sweets. The obese child should be assessed not only in terms of diet but also according to how the parents reinforce the overeating and how the child meets his or her other needs by eating.

Parent-child interactions invariably indicate whether affection is involved in the relationship. The nurse should observe whether the child is listened to and paid attention to or simply told to be quiet and go to the other room. A look at the home will tell the nurse if the parents have adjusted to the child's needs by putting plants and dishes out of reach and have objects for the child to play with. The nurse should observe how much independence the parents allow the child or how fearful they are about the child's urge to explore the world. Are they permissive to the point of danger to the child or are they too restrictive and therefore stifling the child's drives?

The child's behavior toward the parent or the nurse is another indication of whether his or her needs are being met. Children (at least small ones) express their emotions honestly, whereas adults may purposely act more affectionate and accepting toward the child when the nurse is present than they would under normal circumstances.

The experienced nurse is usually familiar with the range of normal behavior for different ages, and if a child's behavior is unusual will often pick it up instantly. This first gut-level reaction may be confirmed after the nurse assesses more details about family interactions. Many experienced nurses report that such initial feelings in most instances do point to problems and should be listened to.

Neglect or abuse can be detected in children even in infancy. In contrast to the happy, smiling, and cooing three-month-old baby who stares at faces intensely and reaches out to strangers, the baby with a blank stare, who avoids eye contact and does not respond with smiles, should arouse the nurse's suspicion. This observation needs to be checked against other observations, however, before conclusions can be drawn, especially since mental retardation may produce similar effects.

As Hollingshead (1941:68) points out, a toddler is driven by a need for acceptance. Extreme behavior, such as aggressive tendencies or constant attention seeking, may point out that such acceptance is or was at one time not available to the extent the child needed it. Some fear of strangers is the norm. Toddlers who cling to the nurse should be regarded as being as unusual as those who are extremely suspicious. Overfriendliness may be a compensation for lack of mothering, whereas suspicion often is a reaction to unfair treatment and abuse.

Older children in dysfunctional families may be shy or have difficulties getting along with other children. They may be rough, irresponsible, or disturbing in school. They may withdraw from others or they may be boastful and try to put themselves in the foreground. Maladjusted children often show psychosomatic symptoms, such as stomachaches, asthma, or headaches, or they may have disturbing symptoms, such as bed-wetting, overeating, or phobias. The nurse should keep in mind that depression in children is often expressed through physical symptoms, but if such symptoms occur, other types of conditions need to be ruled out before conclusions can be drawn.

Teenagers frequently suffer from depression, and the nurse should be particularly aware of the loner who has few friends and does not feel accepted by others. Sometimes this estrangement is due to physical handicaps, but in other cases it derives from psychological problems stemming from the family network.

Adults, too, may show symptoms such as depressed mood, restlessness, complaints about sleeplessness, and compulsive behavior. If such symptoms are picked up by the nurse and the nurse gives the client permission to tell about these troubles, very often the person will take the opportunity to share them.

COMMUNICATION

In Chapter 9 we discussed communication principles as part of the helping relationship. In this chapter our aim is to show the role of communication in family interaction. Nurses skilled in communication techniques are able to use these same principles to assess family communication. For example, a nurse aware of communication blocks between himself or herself and clients will probably observe the same blocks occurring in conversations between family members.

If communication between family members is functional, the relationship between them is more than likely functional also. Dysfunctional communication, on the other hand, strongly suggests difficulties in the relationships. In order for the communication to be functional, it should be sent in a more or less straightforward fashion, and the receiver for the most part needs to be able to interpret the messages correctly. By communicating clearly, the family members can let each other know about themselves and gain understanding and support from others. The sender of messages needs to be aware of roots for possible misunderstandings, such as different connotations of a word or different meanings of words, and the receiver has to clarify messages he or she did not understand before reacting to them.

The communication process is complicated, since it includes not only verbal messages but nonverbal ones as well. Receiving a message is a complex process of first assessing the meaning of the verbal content and then interpreting nonverbal behavior such as gestures, tone of voice, and body language. The receiver next examines the context in which the message was sent, what the sender meant, and what the sender expects from the receiver. This last part of the interpretation is the assessment of the nonverbal content of the message, the hidden message, or what is called *metacommunication.* Satir (1967:76) states that metacommunication is the message about the message. When in Chapter 9 we discussed ways in which the nurse should listen to cues, we were actually talking about assessing metacommunication. Metacommunication may either be verbal or nonverbal, but people cannot communicate without metacommunicating. When person X tells his child that she has done a good job, he metacommunicates to her that he is proud of having her as a daughter. When person Y says, "What a nice day!" she may also mean to say that she is tired of the long winter and that people should get out and enjoy it. Most messages that are sent are in some way incomplete and the receiver is expected to interpret what was not said. At times the sender provides the explanation by giving a verbal metacommunication, such as, "I did not really mean it; it was just a joke," or "I really want you to help me with this."

Assessment of such communication is particularly difficult if there is no congruence between verbal and nonverbal messages. If person X says "I will do this for you" but, instead of smiling, has a slight frown, person Y may well think that he may not really like to do it. The simplest and most functional way to handle such situations, of course, is for the receiver to clarify his or her impression with the sender—for example, "Are you sure that you want to do it? You don't look too happy. Please be honest."

Communication Problems

Problems in communication are often brought on by receivers who have difficulties interpreting sent messages. Not every person is equally skilled in this task. People with consistent problems may get labeled as "paranoid," "depressive," "narcissistic," or "masochistic." People with these conditions selectively interpret messages to "nourish" their psychological problem. The same is true for people who harbor resentment and anger toward the partner of a relationship, and as a result interpret the other's messages according to what they think he or she should be saying rather than what he is actually saying. For example:

HUSBAND: Are you going to wear the yellow dress today? (*Smiles.*)

WIFE: You don't need to tell me what I ought to wear! (*Raising voice*) You rule over my whole life, every inch of me, and I hate it! I don't even feel like going out with you.

HUSBAND: Hey, I'm trying to be *nice*! Lord, it seems like everything I say makes you explode like a bombshell. (*He walks out.*)

The husband may well have meant nothing more than to show interest in his wife's appearance, but, because of past history, his question triggered all kinds of feelings in his wife. First she misinterpreted his smile as being sarcastic, and this made her react angrily to his being "topdog" and ruling over her. Instead of perceiving his message as a simple question, in other words, she felt he really meant to *tell* her—that is, order her—to wear the yellow dress, and so she exploded with resentment.

Communication problems exist not only for the receiver but for the sender as well. Communication is a two-way street in a relationship, and certain patterns are well rehearsed and used repeatedly. As we said before, a good message sender sends messages that are clear and complete; however, sent messages are rarely so complete, since they include nonverbal metacommunication. In addition, all senders send incomplete verbal messages. Dysfunctional senders, however, do this disproportionally often, expecting the receiver to complete the messages for them. Statements such as "You know" or "It's obvious" are parts of incomplete messages. Statements such as "They treat you like a fool!" usually do not specify who "they" are.

Incomplete messages are frequently part of a dysfunctional relationship. Partners who are testing each other tend to assume that the other partner knows their feelings. "He ought to . . . if he loves me," they may say. Instead of saying that she wants an evening out, a wife may tell her husband that her friend Alice really liked a certain show. If her husband responds, "That's good," and continues reading the paper, she will then be disappointed, thinking, "Why can't he see that I need some diversion?" The sender here is convinced that she actually sent a message, but every outsider will recognize that the intended receiver has no choice but to guess what the message means and that, more than likely, he will guess wrong.

The nurse observing such patterns of communication needs to be aware of the frequency with which they happen and the emotional undertones. The nurse should also keep in mind that incomplete messages do not need to be dysfunctional; they are a natural phenomenon, since all messages include a request for validation. In all communication the sender wishes the receiver to agree, to recognize him or her as a worthwhile person. As Satir (1967:73) states, communication is necessarily an incomplete process. Its purpose is to camouflage such requests and prevent the message-sending person from being embarrassed if the receiver does not agree as hoped.

The other difficulty for the community nurse is that clients do not usually openly assume the habitual communication patterns in the nurse's presence, at least during initial sessions. At times children's communication patterns are more indicative of disharmony than the adults' are. Children learn the patterns from their parents. They also learn from the approval or discouragement they receive by sending different kinds of messages. If open verbal messages are not responded to, they will resort to metacommunication, such as attention-getting behavior. If they get scolded for crying, they may resort to feeling sick and being cared for. If they see parents express their anger with insults, they, too, may scream profanities. If parents expect them to obey without question they may start to manipulate their younger siblings to the same end. During child's play some of these communication patterns become clearly visible. Children may show a mother doll and a father doll interacting with each other and use the very same words they have heard previously.

If congruent nonverbal behavior or other indications of dysfunctional communication are observed, the nurse should inform the family members of these observations and discuss with them whether they perceive their interaction to be a problem. The nurse should also be alert to the other extreme, avoidance of communication all together. As long as family members are in physical proximity, they do communicate, even if it is only nonverbally. Certain families, however, avoid communication by physically separating themselves, by staying at work for long hours, by overengaging in activities outside the home. Some families have very little in common, and the members go their own ways. Weekends may be shared with friends rather than with the family. Parents may not know the whereabouts of their children. For this reason, a family assessment ought to include activities that are done together and the time per week the family spends together. Effective communication can occur only if family members are present and willing to share. There should be a mutual commitment for togetherness within the family and communication should be used to understand each other. Changing needs brought on by developmental crises can be met and coped with only if communication channels are kept open. Often the community nurse can work out a time schedule or mutual plan for sharing feelings within the family, but at times problems are deep-seated, and the family needs to be referred to an outside agency for counseling. The community nurse should not hesitate to propose a referral if a need is assessed. This is especially important since too many families referred for marriage counseling have reached a stage at which the extent of damage to their relationship is beyond repair.

REFERENCES

Duvall EM: *Marriage and Family Development.* Philadelphia, Lippincott, 1977.

Epstein L: *Helping People: The Task-Centered Approach.* St. Louis, CV Mosby, 1980.

Hollingshead AB: *Guidance in Democratic Living.* New York, Appleton-Century, 1941.

Jackson DD: The question of family homeostasis. *Psychiatric Quarterly Supplement* 31:79–90, 1957.

Karpman SB: Fairy tales and script drama analysis. *Transactional Analysis Bulletin* 26:39–43, April 1968.

Kempe HC, Helfer RE: *Helping the Battered Child and His Family.* Philadelphia, Lippincott, 1972.

Perls FS: *Gestalt Theory Verbatim.* Lafayette, Calif, Real People Press, 1969.

Reiss D, Oliveri ME: Family paradigm and family coping: A proposal for linking the family's intrinsic adaptive capacities to its responses to stress. *Family Relations* 29:431–444, October 1980.

Satir V; *Conjoint Family Therapy.* Palo Alto, Calif, Science and Behavior Books, 1967.

Walton-Spradley B: *Community Health Nursing: Concepts and Practice.* Boston, Little, Brown, 1981.

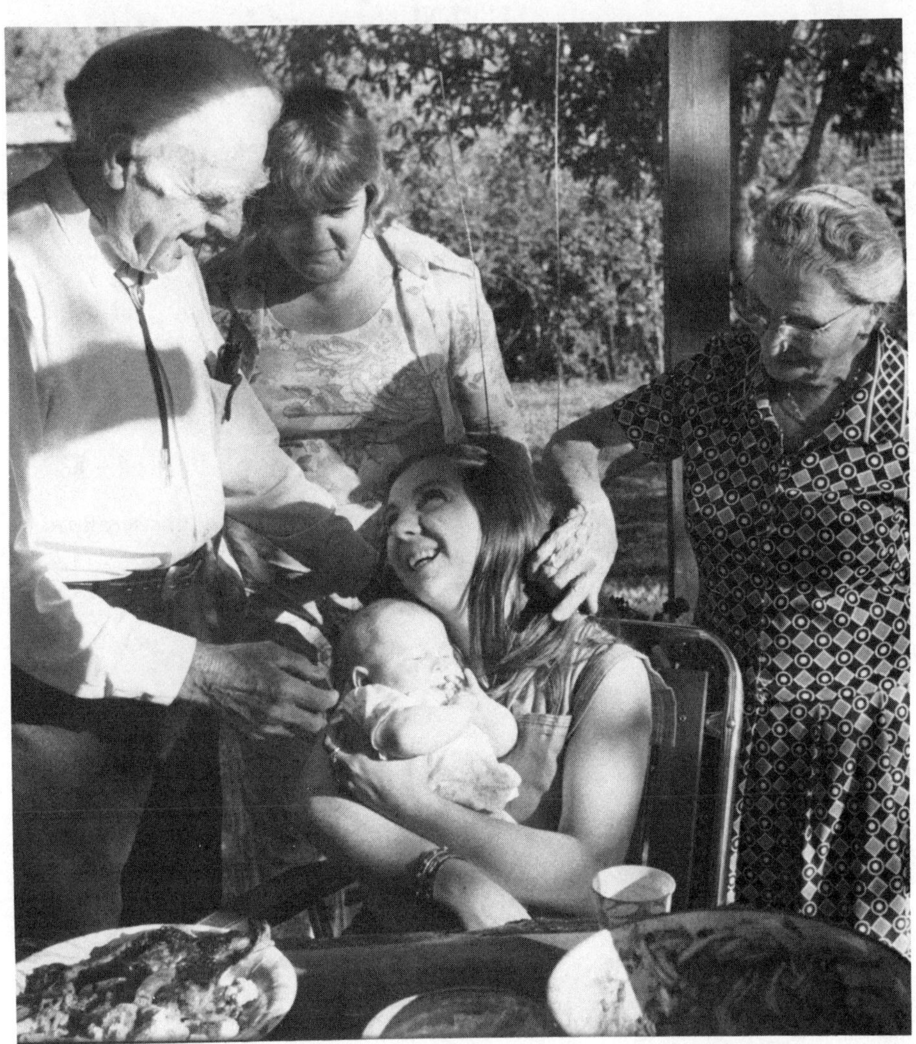

SUZANNE ARMS/JEROBOAM 1980

12

Life-Span Considerations

Just as the individual has to pass through developmental stages such as the ones Erickson (1950) describes, the family, too, can be looked at developmentally. Duval (1977) has developed the widely accepted eight stages of family development:

1. Married couples
2. Childbearing families (oldest child birth–30 months)
3. Families with preschool children (oldest child 2½–6 years)
3. Families with school children (oldest child 6–13 years)
5. Families with teenagers (oldest child 13–20 years)
6. Families launching young adults (first child gone to last child leaving home)
7. Middle-aged parents (empty nest to retirement)
8. Aging family members (retirement to death of both spouses)

Stages 1, 7, and 8 do not include children in the family. The other stages are based on the eldest child's developmental level. Stage 6 is the time when the eldest child is leaving the home. Whereas Erickson's developmental stages are specific to the individual, the family development includes tasks that are mastered by the family as a unit.

Duval's stages are only applicable to the nuclear two-parent family system. This is unfortunate since today atypical families are on the rise. However, a nurse who understands the development of the nuclear family can easily transfer certain aspects to one-parent families, extended families, single adult families, and so on. The relationship of a married couple may be more intimate than the platonic relationship of two adults sharing a household, but the two arrangements have many characteristics in common.

STAGE 1: MARRIED COUPLES

This stage is likely to be the most important stage with regard to the family's success in passing through its life cycle. As discussed in Chapter 11, family interaction problems or communication problems often have their roots in the marital relationship. The task the two people are faced with is the establishment of a mutually satisfying relationship, which includes emotional and sexual satisfaction. Marriage today is still glorified by our society, and (in spite of hard evidence to the contrary) young people in love believe they have found a partner for life. Once the wedding is over and the couple sets into an everyday routine, they suddenly realize that the person they married has some peculiar habits they never noticed before and interests other than in the spouse and lovemaking. The partners also realize that they now have responsibilities such as rent, bills, grocery shopping, household chores they may or may not have been familiar with prior to the marriage.

The couple's friendship circle also changes, and they may no longer feel comfortable with the singles groups they previously associated with. Instead they may need to find a new identity and new friends. Both partners need to sacrifice close bonds with their parents and gain increased independence. They are now in need of each other's support more than ever before.

Reorganization of their lifestyle also needs to occur. They have to decide how to earn and spend money, to find satisfying ways of spending leisure time together, to meet social obligations with an extended family twice the size as before. They need to start setting goals for the future, agree on whether or not to have children, discuss birth control.

Kahn (1981:135–137) lists the basic elements for a marital relationship as *communication, sharing,* and *cooperation.* Let us consider these.

Communication

A young couple must communicate openly from the beginning of their marriage. The task becomes more difficult if they do not share their struggles and doubts, if they misinterpret each other's messages or are distrustful of or dishonest with each other. If hard feelings are created in an argument, they should be talked about and interpreted. If such feelings cannot be released, they are likely to create more anger and resentment and influence the interpretation of communication.

Intervening factors in forming a communicative relationship include past history, lack of role models practicing effective communication, and psychological problems and resulting unwillingness to share. People with a poor self-image often do not willingly share how they feel and think, since they are afraid that the partner may reject them.

The sexual relationship is another form of communication. A relationship that provides mutual pleasure and satisfaction also communicates acceptance, whereas sexual rejection is usually taken seriously by the partner and interpreted as rejection of him or her as a person. If a person tries to please the partner, it helps to bind the whole relationship; if a person has sexual intercourse only for selfish enjoyment, the lack of caring is readily conveyed to the partner.

The sexual relationship as well as the total marital relationship needs to develop and deepen over time. Unless both partners feel a commitment to work together toward constantly improving the relationship and overcoming problems and difficulties, they are likely not to succeed. Communication is the key to such success.

Sharing

Sharing is related to communication in that it can only occur effectively if communication is established. Sharing includes not only the material possessions brought into the marriage but more importantly experiences good and bad, relationships with friends, the extended family, and later on the children.

In many marriages, sharing of financial resources becomes a conflict. Partners with different values, likes, and dislikes may not agree on how to save or spend money. Unless they find ways to compromise and give in, however, bitterness and anger toward each other will grow and spread to other areas, until the couple will feel there is nothing left between them and that the love they started out with is gone as well.

A functional couple spends time together and finds common interests. Experiences that both can get excited about together are the best ones. Separate experiences should be shared so that they may learn from each other.

Cooperation

The third area on Kahn's list, cooperation carries the concept of sharing somewhat further. Cooperation is doing work together to make the relationship function. Managing the home, for instance, includes tasks that are not always pleasurable; the couple should discuss and agree upon a labor division acceptable to both. Social and recreational activities should also be a product of mutual planning. Without agreement, confusion and friction is likely to result. It is easy to see that here, too, communication plays an important part.

If these three areas are mastered satisfactorily, the couple will begin to accept a new identity through which they see themselves no longer as two individuals but as a unit that makes them both stronger and happier.

Community health nurses are frequently not in the position to help a newly married couple complete their task, since these clients as a rule do not show up in visiting nurse agencies until there are babies in the family. Community nurses working in places such as family-planning clinics, private doctors' offices, and outpatient clinics should invest some of their energy in teaching these young people. Teaching in groups is extremely effective, where several couples may be helped to recognize that everyone has initial problems and that there are ways to work these problems out and find solutions. This arrangement may also help start to establish a support system by building friendships between couples in the group. The nurse who is aware of potential problems and uses empathy and skills in the group process will be truly instrumental in preventing failure in marriage, broken hearts, and unhappy children.

STAGE 2: CHILDBEARING FAMILIES

For many couples the time when the first baby is born turns out to be very stressful and difficult. Ideally the couple should wait to have a first child until their relationship has established open communication channels and mutual respect and affection in spite of differences. Problems invariably arise for couples who believe the solution to their differences is to have a baby to create interests in common and bring them back together. Young people need to realize that a baby brings conflict, stress, and demands for personal sacrifice. Unless the marital relationship rests on a solid foundation, a child will increase the stress and friction, and situations will arise of the type discussed in Chapter 11.

Having a baby is another area in which societal values and the media have created romanticized expectations among parents-to-be. Future mothers dream about holding a cuddly baby in their arms and rocking him to sleep. The pronoun "him" is used here purposefully, for even today most mothers-to-be wish their first child to be a boy and show at least a little disappointment if it does not turn out that way. The disappointment is even greater if the girl baby cries for four hours every night, turns stiff in the mother's arms instead of wanting to be cuddled, and refuses to go to sleep until seven in the morning. The husband may find himself abruptly awakened by his sobbing wife, who can no longer handle the situation; whether he supports her or blows up depends, of course, on his temperament.

The greater the discrepancy between parental expectations and infant reality, the greater the stress on the parents. Even the best baby requires the parents' adjustment to the feeding and diaper changing, so that the household routine will suddenly come to revolve around the newborn. Some initial exhaustion of the parents is to be expected, especially if they do not get help from a grandmother or friend during the first weeks.

If the couple has a firmly established relationship and mutual support, they will be able to absorb the initial stress and to start to enjoy the baby. Once the infant smiles and responds to them, their efforts will seem rewarded and they will feel that the first troubles were worthwhile.

Here, too, community health nurses can soften the blow by good anticipatory guidance, perhaps offered in combination with tips mothers can use to solve baby problems. Young people do not usually change their minds about wanting the child if they have a better idea of what it will be like. Group teaching is extremely helpful. Bringing a new mother and father into the group who can tell about their experiences is likely to have a lasting effect on the expectant couples. Anticipatory guidance should cover not only the process of labor, childbirth methods, and child care but also emotional aspects and methods for dealing with stress.

Even when the child is part of the family and the parents fairly adjusted to the new routine, the couple still needs to grow into their new roles as parents. Moreover, the family unit must find a new identity, for relationships now involve not only the parents but the child as well. In order to allow for nurturing relationships between child and mother and child and father, the basic marital relationship has to be firm. As we discussed in Chapter 11, the child cannot meet needs that the parents do not meet with each other. On the contrary, such needs become intensified if the child is placed in the middle.

The father must allow his wife to form a firm and loving relationship with the baby, even though it means her attention will no longer be focused solely on her husband. Frequently some temporary jealousy of the husband is the result. Mothers unwilling to share the baby with the father will intensify this feeling to the point where the father will feel left out. In many modern families, fathers take part in the experience of preparing for the baby, in labor and delivery, and later in caring for it.

Mothers, too, may encounter difficulties adjusting to their new role. Many women with newborn babies feel socially isolated after the initial excitement is over, for they can no longer go out as they please. Women who have been professionally active or involved in many social activities are especially apt to feel lonely during the long hours the baby sleeps. Going out in evenings may be harder as well, since a very young baby cannot be entrusted to an inexperienced babysitter.

This is a stage at which the marriage should be solidified, for the partners will need each other more than ever. The new baby can be an immense gratification, but only if the two parents are able to mutually share it and adjust to its changing needs. While the child sleeps many hours at first, as it gets older it needs more attention. The parents need to be concerned with its growth and stimulation, safety, and health.

Couples with new babies may be visited by nurses or seen by nurse practitioners in doctors' offices, well-baby clinics, or immunization clinics. Community nurses find innumerable opportunities for teaching baby care, safety measures, disease prevention, nutrition, growth and development, and anticipation of needs the child will have as it grows older. Such teaching can be done both individually and in groups. Nurses are not likely to find more attentive learners than young mothers and fathers. Questions about baby care—how to handle colic, diarrhea, fever, diaper rash, and so on—may seem endless. Anxiety in young parents is great. Mothers often need help with nursing their babies, or nursing mothers may be afraid their infants are undernourished. Telling them that they have a healthy-looking baby may offer immediate relief.

Although mothers need to be advised on how to go about caring for their babies, nurses need to make sure the information the mothers have collected from other sources does not conflict with new information. Conflicting information can be devastating to insecure parents, for it not only leaves them confused, it also undermines the relationship with the nurse. Teaching needs to be adjusted to what mothers already know and their understanding of advice obtained elsewhere.

Besides anxiety, insecurity is probably new parents' greatest problem, for the first baby is an "experiment." Every baby is different, and for many problems there are no clear-cut rules that will work for all. Mothers therefore need to get to know the baby's personality and study its reactions to different approaches. Nurses can only suggest possible ways to tackle a problem (such as a baby's refusing to eat vegetables) and the mother must pick out what way works best for her baby.

Community nurses should keep in mind that mothers many times know best, even if they have no formal education. After all, they have spent a great deal of time observing every reaction of the baby and know it better than anyone else. Nurses also need to realize that giving parents credit for their good work with the baby works best in establishing a good relationship with them. To get off on the right foot, the nurse should initially focus on the parents and their needs and express empathy and understanding of the problems a new baby creates. This inquiring about their welfare and finding out if their needs are met tells the parents that the nurse is concerned for the family as a whole. Whatever parents do well should be pointed out first; aspects that need improvement will consequently more likely be accepted.

Since parents generally are more receptive to health teaching during this stage of their life, home visits or clinic visits are an excellent opportunity for the nurse to assess and teach primary prevention for the whole family. The nurse can stress the importance of such teaching by pointing out that a happy and healthy child needs a happy and healthy family. There are not many parents who are not concerned about the child's health and happiness.

STAGE 3: FAMILIES WITH PRESCHOOL CHILDREN

The child's becoming mobile brings great changes to the lifestyle of the family. Mothers who have found deep satisfaction in the symbiotic relationship with their children are now asked to let them go. The children will want independence and will let the parents know unmistakably, endlessly taxing the parents' nerves. With boundless energy they will explore their world—the parents' house—which often will create severe conflicts of interest. The child may want to smash eggs to watch what comes out of the shells, while the mother wrings her hands.

Safety measures are imperative in the house at this point. Community nurses need to instruct parents how to "child-proof" the home but still allow the children opportunities to explore in order to let them develop to their full potential. A tour around the house by nurse and parents is helpful in assessing possible hazards such as poisons, steep stairs, and open windows.

Another of the child's needs at this period of life is a need for limits. Healthy discipline needs to emerge and the parents need to establish their roles in meeting this responsibility (see Chapter 11). Communication channels need to be kept open in order to discuss these limits, which should give the child enough freedom to grow but which prevent danger. Both parents need to be comfortable with the limits and agree to enforce them consistently.

Family routine needs to be such that young children's physical needs are met. They need a routine; the day needs to be structured so that they can anticipate events such as naps and rest periods. Because the children's nutritional needs are changing, the parents should be flexible enough to let them experiment with finger foods and later with spoon and fork as a learning experience and as a way of fostering acceptance of a greater variety of foods.

Even though children may be the center of the family, the parents have other concerns as well, of course, such as financial stability and career. The mother may reenter the work world and leave the child in a day-care center or with a babysitter. Values concerning the family will be forming, and the parents must start to consider the future, for the child will have increasing needs as time goes on. The parents need to assess their responsibilities not only to provide material goods but also to meet all family members' needs for emotional support, affection, and security. If more children are born into the family, there must be readjustment to allow for more than one growing individual. More space may be needed, which involves moving to a different home and different neighborhood. The parents may also visualize themselves as being part of the community, so that, besides the work place, they may be active in organizations such as the church, preschool, clubs, and political groups.

Community nurses are often involved with families of preschoolers. This family-life stage includes many areas of teaching. Safety, sibling rivalry, nutrition, what to look for when choosing a babysitter, growth and development and expectation of future growth and development are just a few. One of the most important areas to assess is coping skills. How do the parents cope with the stress imposed on them by the child's development needs? How does that stress compare to stress from external sources? How does the quality of the marital relationship intervene with imposed stress?

Psychological problems often interfere with the efficiency of parenting in this period. Mothers who are not sure of themselves and have a low self-image will resent the child's testing their willpower. Children in their twos are especially hard to handle. Insecure mothers may fear that they are losing control over the child. They may also resent having to share the child with the world. The gratification the baby provided them with through complete trust and acceptance is lost. They may find it again with a new baby, but they may not be able to satisfy the first child's needs, especially if he or she acts up owing to the presence of a new brother or sister. Mothers who cling to their preschoolers—who overprotect them, do not let them experiment, and prevent them from growing up emotionally—may cause much harm to themselves and the children.

Nurses who recognize the difficulties of this stage can assist parents in adjusting to these changes by listening to their concerns, by giving them confidence in pointing out their strengths and the child's healthy development, by helping them to look at the child's behavior as a "stage" that will not last, and by working out with them ways they can meet the child's needs without sacrificing their own.

STAGE 4: FAMILIES WITH SCHOOL CHILDREN

The first day of school for their eldest child comes as a shock to some parents. It means a big step away from parental control. The parents now have to share the child with the community. The child will learn and accept values that are beyond the parents' control. He or she will thus no longer be a product of the family only. Parents who have difficulties are usually the same ones who resented the arrival of the toddler stage.

Communication patterns in the healthy family should now include the children more and more in verbal discussions. They are becoming individuals and should be respected and protected within the family. They need to share their experiences with their parents and siblings. Many families complain about their school-age children being "mouthy" and rebellious. Parents who have set strict limits and rules and who have firmly allocated tasks within the household may find it difficult to maintain them. The children are now exposed to the community. They discover how other people live, and they have a keen sense of privileges that other children have and they do not. They start questioning the parents' values and attitudes, rebel against restrictions such as a small allowance or a set bedtime that does not seem fair since everyone else goes to bed later. They demand explanations and reasons for restrictions and argue endlessly, until parents either give in or lose their tempers. Manipulating parents becomes a great sport. The children strive for a sense of power within the family, and if the family reacts by increased suppression, they are likely to start a small-scale guerrilla war.

The best way out of this dilemma is to relax the rules as much as can be done safely. Children overestimate their ability to make coherent judgments and may feel the consequences of their actions if the parents relax too much. Ten-year-olds who are allowed to decide on their own bedtimes, for example, may well read till late at night and be tired and inattentive in school on the next day. Rules should be set, but they should make sense. Family discussions held for the purpose of explaining these rules may be exhausting and tedious for parents, but they are important.

The school-age stage determines to a large extent how the teenage stage will turn out. Parents who do not communicate with their children are now likely to lose them, for they have begun to relate to their friends and tune out the parents. Very restrictive rules and regulations are not the norm in our society, and excessively restrictive parents may sooner or later suffer the consequences. Children may react by becoming distrustful and by pulling away from the family, or by cutting themselves off from their friends and the mainstream of society. Either way the children's self-esteem will be negatively affected because they will no longer be accepted by the family or because they have failed to validate themselves among their peers.

The battle for independence used to be a characteristic of the teenage years. Today the storm starts sooner; the so-called "latency period" is no longer quiet. Because parents tend to compare their children to themselves as they were brought up and tend to stick to old values, they need to be helped to adjust to changing norms. The key to this, again, is communication. Good communication is effective not only in facilitating the difficult process of adjusting limits, but it also leads to rewarding family relationships.

Today's children are able to think and to question not only family rules but also the world around them. Parents who are able to listen are also able to enjoy them. They can discuss human behavior, world happenings, or the phenomena of science or nature with the children and help them understand. As time goes on, parents can facilitate the children's growth, but at the same time they, too, will grow and enjoy a fresh approach and new outlook on problems. Their relationship with the children can become one of mutual understanding, respect, and affection rather than one of the powerful suppressing the weak.

Community nurses need to have a clear understanding of the changes occurring in today's families and the larger society. They need to recognize the discrepancies between societal norms and family values and pinpoint the nature of the consequent friction the family experiences. Nurses can do a great deal of good by supporting the parents' concern for their children and recognizing their strengths. Many parents faced with the tasks of this stage in the family life cycle are as insecure as when they had a new baby. The adjustment is difficult since they cannot draw on past role models from their own childhoods. Again, many of these problems can be solved in discussion and sharing groups. Since there are no role models in the past, parents must find support among themselves. Nothing helps more than finding out that these problems are shared by other families.

Community nurses who have lived through this stage themselves will undoubtedly be the best group leaders. However, other nurses can be effective as long as they are careful to avoid giving unsolicited advice, especially in group situations, where parents are quick to say, "How do you know? You never had to raise kids!" The role of the nurse is not to provide solutions but to raise questions for members of the group to examine so that they can arrive at their own solutions.

The same holds true for individual counseling. The best a nurse can do is give examples of how other families have handled the same problems and let the family being counseled decide whether or not they want to try the same approach. The most important part of the helping relationship is trust, which is most effectively established by the nurse's recognizing the family's strengths and building on them. It must be remembered that an insecure family first needs to know that they are doing something right; they will then cooperate in trying to correct things they do wrong.

STAGE 5: FAMILIES WITH TEENAGERS

The teenage stage is often thought of as a totally new phenomenon that hits the family all of a sudden. This is not so. The family's success in negotiating this stage is related to their success in several previously discussed areas. The first area is discipline. Whereas limits need to be narrow and firm for children in preschool years, they should become gradually more relaxed until adolescence, when the young person is expected to handle many important decisions independently and no longer needs the parents' limits setting. The second area, communication, on the other hand, needs to expand from the stage where cooperation is demanded to a communication between almost equals, a give-and-take process that leads to mutual growth.

The third area of growth is trust. Initially, trust is rather one-sided. Everyone knows that toddlers cannot be trusted, but young children need to trust their parents for optimal development. As the children learn and internalize limits and values, the parents can trust them more and more. First they can be let alone for short periods without pulling the cat's tail or defoliating the plants. Later they can be allowed to play outside when Mother is confident that they will not run away. School-age children can be depended on to perform their duties independently and may watch the house for short periods of time. Teenagers need to be trusted to make their own decisions. Some of these decisions are extremely important and carry consequences that will be felt all during later life, such as career decisions or sexual behavior.

Children need to be trusted in order to develop self-esteem. A mother who believes that her children are able to be responsible and get their homework done will convey to them that she trusts them. They in turn will respond to this attitude by showing her that they actually can. As previously mentioned, the process should start very early and it should be accompanied by rewards. Children need to be rewarded for positive behavior. They then feel recognized and become self-confident as they are told that they can do it. Since their parents trust them, they will not disappoint them.

Expectations have to be reasonable, however. Transgressions and occasional abuse of such trust need to be expected. Children react positively to parents who reprimand them for having violated their unwritten contract with the parents and hurt their feelings. Children should be told that in order to maintain such trust they need to live up to it. If, on the other hand, parents react with anger, revenge, and subsequent mistrust, they leave the child with guilt feelings, decreased self-esteem, and the belief that he or she is not able to fulfill this expectation.

It can be easily seen that trust and communication go hand in hand. Communication needs to include the parents' being open and honest about their own emotions. They need to communicate early on how the child's behavior affects them. Children need to know when they make them angry or what aspects of their behavior make them sad. Only then can the children learn to respect others and be considerate of other people's needs, and only then can they respect themselves.

It is a sad fact that a deficiency in this process of communication leading to mutual respect cannot be easily repaired after symptoms show up in the teenage stage. Damaged self-esteem, anger, hostility, feelings of worthlessness, drifting without goals, living without purpose, rebelling against society, seeking comfort among one's own kind, being involved in dysfunctional or delinquent behavior are just a few of the detrimental symptoms that are rooted in this process. The community nurse thus has a great responsibility here. No nurse should consider a family beyond help. Every effort should be made to improve relationships within families. It is probably the most worthwhile endeavor a helping person can strive for.

Teenagers who are victims of dysfunctional families need intervention that goes beyond the nurse's capabilities in most cases. Even then, the outcome is doubtful. Family therapy may be helpful, but it is a long, expensive process and the results may be unavailing in families with severe problems. Often young people are better off if they are helped to separate from the family and gain self-esteem by way of a new self-image as independent persons. Peer groups may be the most effective medium for change, and community nurses who are comfortable working with this age group can be very effective. Adolescents need support. They need someone to listen to them and understand them so that they can value themselves.

Community nurses working with families are effective in helping the fairly functional family adjust to new challenges. Often parents are troubled by the sexual maturity of their children. Again, this conflict stems from changes in societal values, which may clash with the values of many individual families. However, if the family members communicate well in other areas, it is possible that the nurse as intermediator can bring them together to share their feelings and opinions and to gain understanding of each other's needs.

Other areas of frequent conflict are over independence and relaxation of parental restrictions. Often a family will acquiesce to the young person's requests and the teenager will abuse it by engaging in unacceptable acts such as drug use, sexual behavior, or poor study habits. The community nurse at times may prove invaluable in averting a disaster by bringing the delinquent and the rest of the family back together and by getting them to realize they actually care about each other's well-being. The key to this is the helping relationship—that is, learning to listen and respect each member's point of view and to make one's own point of view understandable to other family members.

In summary, the teenage stage is a culmination of all other tasks the family has dealt with during previous stages. Communication becomes sorely tested, and stability and cooperation within the family is rocked on many occasions. The family needs to support its growing young people, allow them some leeway for experimentation without being condemned, and let them learn by making mistakes within limits. The family also needs to support new interests and goals of its adolescents and let them find their identity outside the family. Parents need to understand the adolescent's urge to separate and recognize that any effort of the family to prevent this will be vigorously attacked.

STAGE 6: FAMILIES LAUNCHING YOUNG ADULTS

Letting sons and daughters go on to begin their own lives is difficult for all parents who have invested their emotional energy in them. A deep loss is felt, and some grieving is likely to take place. This stage is particularly hard for mothers who have devoted their entire lives to the children and for whom, once the children leave, their purpose in life has disappeared. Moreover, the further away the children move geographically, the harder it is for the parents to maintain close contact with them.

The change in our society toward more mobility makes this stage more difficult to bear. In times past, by the time the last child had left the home, several grandchildren had arrived to populate the home base. With the new generation staying in the same town, home became a second home for grandchildren and a new purpose in life for the grandparents. Today couples have fewer children, and chances are slimmer that they will stay within the same community. During the launching stage, therefore, the parents need to prepare themselves emotionally for abrupt change.

Ideally there should be a shift of values or priorities. Professional or career goals may become more important in many families. Wives may educate themselves for a second career, or a couple may intensify their interests in recreational activities or community functions, activities that may lead to more sharing and a deeper relationship.

However, problems may arise in families in which the wife fails to acquire her own identity, perhaps because she does not have the self-confidence to try something new, since she has not achieved anything that earned her respect within the community besides raising children. The problems may be especially severe if the husband gets more absorbed in his career and work responsibilities. The wife may end up left out and bored, without any goals for herself. Again, the success in this stage greatly depends on the basic relationship between the original partners. As time goes on and fewer of their needs can be taken care of by the children, dependence on each other becomes greater. If both partners are equally dependent upon each other, they are likely to be equally willing to take care of each other's needs. However, problems arise if one of them—in most cases the wife—becomes more dependent while the other partner's lifestyle does not allow for such dependency.

Community nurses need to work individually with the family member affected most by the change and help him or her find new goals and a new outlook on life. If the problem lies within the marital relationship, the partner should be encouraged to join the sessions, so that the nurse can aim at improving communication. The partners should disclose their needs to each other in order to find ways to adjust. They may find they have to allow more time for each other or common goals and activities. This is only possible, however, if their relationship is based on concern and affection. A referral should be considered if hard feelings and resentment are expressed about the relationship.

STAGE 7: MIDDLE-AGED PARENTS

Since people are getting older and having fewer children, the time marriage partners spend together with just each other is on the increase. A new trend, however, indicates that many couples postpone having children for some time after getting married, which brings them to a more advanced stage of their life by the time the children leave the house and thus shortens the middle-aged parents stage. This presents another problem. Whereas women who finish their child-rearing duties at an early age still have the chance to engage in a new career, for late starters in their fifties such a change is more problematic.

The middle-age crisis mostly occurs in women, but it can also hit men, though usually at a somewhat later age. Depression may set in when a woman realizes her youth is lost and her parental task is done. The future may seem nothing to look forward to, bringing only loneliness and loss of agility, beauty, and health. Many women react to this crisis by engaging in radical changes. Quiet people start to socialize more. Housewives go back to school. Many such individuals have the feeling that time is running out and that if they are to achieve anything in life they have to do it now.

The community nurse's role in this situation is one of support. A nurse can help the client evaluate whether the plans are realistic and what the future will look like after such a change is completed. Some women also need an estimate of the effort they need to put into such a change, in order to judge whether or not they will be able to withstand the stress. They also need to consider how such a change will affect their marriage partner, and the partner should be in full support of the endeavor.

People who lack the energy to make changes and who let themselves be overcome by depression may or may not react to the nurse's encouragement. The nurse should concentrate on helping them to boost their self-esteem by realizing their potential and their strengths. If this is not possible, a referral is needed. Groups concentrating on women's problems or assertiveness training may be beneficial to some individuals. The nurse needs to assess the root of their depression carefully and determine whether the condition is in fact only a simple reaction to diverse losses or if its basis is deeper seated within the person's personality.

Men are less frequently visible to the community health nurse. Industrial nurses who work for employers may see such clients, usually at the point where their health is failing. Often their main source of stress is work related rather than family related; however, much of the stress results from frustration about getting older and worry over having "missed the boat" in their careers. They may have had high professional aspirations that were never realized. Coming home to a family without children and to a wife who suffers from depression may intensify such frustration. The man's home may then serve as an everyday reminder that the best part of his life is over.

Marriages that have been reasonably stable may crumble at this point. It is imperative that the two partners learn to accept the unavoidable, the aging process. A woman may be able to escape it temporarily by engaging in a new career, or either marriage partner may engage in a love affair with a younger person in order to feel rejuvenated; however, the fact of aging remains.

STAGE 8: AGING FAMILY MEMBERS

Whereas during the middle-aged parents stage the married couple has to get reacquainted and readjusted to each other once the children have left home, during the final stage of life such adjustment is even more needed. Once retirement begins, the couple finds they have a lot of time on hand, and if the relationship is not stable, the constant togetherness can create friction and hostility. The difficulties may be accelerated by the retiring person's emotional problems. Retirement is a difficult step for many people who have felt useful and fulfilled within their jobs. Moreover, jobs provide not only something to do but also the opportunity to socialize and feel part of a group. At retirement, people realize that the group can function without them, that their ties with the people remaining on the job are weakened, and that it is harder to replenish their self-esteem without achievement through the job. People who do not have interests and projects they can tackle with enthusiasm and that will provide a sense of achievement similar to their previous work will likely have difficulties adjusting—and their being in a depressed mood will affect their partner's emotional well-being.

The first task, then, is adjusting to a totally new lifestyle. Depending on the support of the extended family, this change may be more or less successful. Living quarters may need to be changed. Often the original home is too big, and cleaning becomes too great a task. The couple may want to get involved in new friendships with other retired people and find new activities that both partners can share. Grandchildren may provide a sense of satisfaction and joy and a feeling that their life has been useful.

The next task is a change in outlook on life. Whereas a young person lives primarily in the present and works toward a future, the old person's future is less promising. Health is deteriorating, friends are passing away, body function is reduced, and many interests and activities can no longer be pursued. Adjustment to aging is therefore a process of starting to derive satisfaction from little things in the present, such as grandchildren's visits, a walk around the block, or presence of a pet, and of maintaining the ego not by new achievements, but by drawing strength from accomplishments in the past. Accomplishment of this task provides a feeling of having lived a good life and now deserving a rest and some last enjoyment before making room for the new generation to continue their work. Ideally this should not be resignation or giving up but acceptance of the unavoidable accompanied by personal satisfaction and spiritual growth. Resulting wisdom and strength can be a source of inspiration to the young.

This youth-oriented society has destroyed much of the beauty of old age. It is difficult for old people to gain a sense of accomplishment if the world around them sends the message that they are really no good any more and that it would be better and cheaper if they no longer existed. Elderly couples often live by themselves, removed from the young generation, because they do not want to be a burden. Becoming ill and debilitated may damage the spirit, for our society stresses that one should be strong, fit, and independent in order to accomplish tasks for the good of everyone. As a result, the elderly may experience depression and loneliness.

Some couples attempt to postpone the inevitable by "feeling young" and pretending that nothing has changed. They live in retirement settlements removed from the young, who constantly remind them of their age, denying reality until disaster strikes. Or they belong to clubs, go to parties, and try to live it up. Still others fight back by being involved in community activities, political action, social projects, or other worthwhile activities that provide them with a sense of accomplishment. However, these, too, are only temporary solutions, if the task of accepting one's fate is not completed at the same time.

The loss of one's mate is likely to be the greatest test of inner strength. Many individuals never fully recover from this blow, especially if they do not have a supportive extended family and cannot find a purpose in continuing to live. Religion may provide such a purpose; indeed, religion is probably the best facilitator of the aging process. However, many individuals do not have this resource and need to find inner strength elsewhere.

Community health nurses are frequently involved with the elderly. Failing health brings old people to clinics and hospitals, and often they need visits at home. They may be required to adjust to special diet regimes or other supportive health measures, and the nurse has to teach them how to go about making these changes. By doing a complete assessment, the nurse may detect the difficulties in adjusting to old age. Nurses will frequently encounter depression and loneliness. In fact, depression in old age is so common that it is considered to be the norm rather than the exception. Community health nurses, however, should realize that depression can be avoided, and they will no doubt visit some individuals who radiate a sense of joy and serenity that often leaves a lasting impression. One example is the 98-year-old woman who said, "I enjoy getting up every day and seeing the sun come up, and I enjoy my great-grandchildren visiting me on the weekend. My one goal is to live to be 99, but if God calls me, it's all right, I'm ready."

The most effective community health nurse is the one who not only teaches the elderly but is willing to learn from them. Old people are a wonderful resource for the nurse herself to learn from in order to grow personally and spiritually. Society has impoverished the young population by removing the old. The elderly have learned about the nature of life over many years. They have had experiences and lived through times that are foreign to the young, although society makes them believe that what they have learned has no value and that their experiences have no more relevance. Community nurses should know better. Whoever has listened to old tales knows how exciting these stories are and how much can be learned. Many stories are eye openers. Young people forget that life has not always been the way it is now. The old stories let them realize how the world is changing and see what the old generation has contributed in order to make life what it is today. The stories help one to get a new outlook on life, to see it in the historical perspective, and to recognize where young persons stand in the development of present-day events. By placing themselves in the flow of time and recognizing the direction in which they are going, they are able to gain a new identity.

Old people often are not aware of the value of their sharing the past with younger people. Community nurses should therefore show interest and listen to them. They should learn from them and express to them what they have learned so that they will begin to value their own resources.

Some community nurses are active in programs that help seniors to use their talents, such as participating in grandparent programs in nursery schools and kindergartens. Many of these programs involving senior citizens are excellent devices for lifting old people's spirits and letting them realize their potential. However, nurses need to be aware of old people's need to come to terms with their futures and to use caution in suggesting involvement in activities that serve to increase denial and provide escape from reality. In short, nurses are most helpful if they are willing to listen, since giving the elderly a chance to be teachers is truly therapeutic and is nourishing self-esteem more than any other nursing intervention.

THE ATYPICAL FAMILY

Duval's (1977) framework focuses only on the nuclear family, as we noted; however, nonnuclear families have become more frequent in our society. Unfortunately, no conceptual framework has been suggested for other than the nuclear family. This part of the chapter attempts to point out some differences and some common characteristics between the nuclear family and other arrangements.

The One-Parent Family

This family is probably the one most frequently encountered after the nuclear family, but the developmental stages by which families become this type varies. Some single mothers never get married and assume their responsibilities independently at the time the baby is born. Or they may live with their parents initially and become independent later. Other families—the greatest percentage—become one-parent families owing to divorce. Some families go through series of substitute fathers or mothers, and some end by reconverting into a nuclear family, often with a mixed set of children.

There is no specific set of problems or tasks that needs to be mastered by one-parent families, since these problems depend on the individual nature of each family.

As pointed out earlier, the essential characteristic of the nuclear family is the marital relationship of the two partners and the fact that they are able to meet each other's needs. Keeping this in mind, it is obvious that the one-parent family encounters special difficulties. The widowed or divorced single parent has lost the most obvious, natural source of meeting his or her needs, so that any stress and tension get transferred to the children. In addition, in reaction to the loss suffered, the single parent often modifies the relationship with the children. For instance, if a child has previously been siding with both parents and considered it to be his or her responsibility to hold the partners together, a divorce will make the child feel guilty. As a result, a son will feel obligated to "take care" of his mother—and often the mother welcomes this opportunity to fulfill her own needs. However, since the mother has other needs, sexual needs, which the son cannot meet, if another man enters the picture, the son is apt to have a strong reaction. Afraid of being left out, feeling deprived, he again will feel that he has failed, since he could not keep his mother happy. Fathers and daughters go through similar problems, and the problem even occurs with a parent and same-sex child, although the motive is somewhat different: the child goes through a process of identification with the same-sex parent but feels strong emotional ties to the other parent, which are reinforced by the fear of losing that parent as well. Having to share the parent with another adult again is perceived as a further loss.

Nurses who assess such families need first to explore how the single parents meet their needs. Sometimes an extended family helps to ease the blow of separation or divorce to the parent and the child. Children who have felt close to their grandparents will have some stability in their lives, and by sharing the children with the grandparents, the parent minimizes the danger of overdependence in the parent-child relationship. If there is no extended family, a single parent needs to look outside the family for people to help meet his or her needs.

To get a clear picture, the nurse should assess if the parent participates in social functions, belongs to any groups, or has friends she can trust. The children, too, should be assessed as to how they relate to peers and get along in school. The nurse should find out how well the children have worked through their grief about losing a parent and whether they can relate to other adults who can serve as role models. This last point is especially important for a child living with a parent of opposite sex.

The nurse should realize that children in a divorced family are not necessarily emotionally damaged or maladjusted. Often, in fact, children who work through the divorce successfully end up being better able to cope with future problems. A healthy parent-child relationship should be warm and loving. The two should have time to spend with each other, but give each other the opportunity to be alone and the freedom to associate with other people.

A single-parent family with more than one child functions in much the same way as a single-parent family with only one child. A dysfunctional parent may make one of the children a substitute for the former marital partner, and as a result this child will not only have difficulties functioning in the outside world but be put into a difficult position vis-à-vis other siblings. The functional family, too, looks for support on the outside.

The single parent needs to pass through much of the same life cycle as the two-parent family, except that the single person lacks the support of an intimate partner. Such a parent is likely to experience the greatest need for support when the first baby is born. It is difficult worrying not only about the baby's care but also about how to provide financially. Single parents who have no extended family backing them up with money, baby-sitting, and the like, are likely to experience a great deal of stress. They may have to apply for public assistance, stop going to school, and find babysitters willing to care for infants. Young mothers may end up overwhelmed by the unexpected responsibilities.

Many community health nurses are involved with unwed mothers, first helping them regulate their daily routines, later helping them make plans for the future. A community nurse can help the mother accept her baby by showing her how to solve baby-care problems and how to make mothering a rewarding experience. The nurse can show the mother who her baby is and how much it can do and understand even as a newborn, can make her feel good about her ability to take care of it, and can provide guidance as to the joys and troubles she should expect in the future. Since mothering is a difficult task in today's society, the nurse should remain available to the young mother even after the first crises are past, giving her help with further tasks such as planning for economic security, finding role models for the child, obtaining the best child care, and learning to communicate with the child. Moreover, a young mother needs to be helped to grow emotionally and find ways to fulfill her own needs. Much learning can be accomplished in groups, and such referrals should be highly encouraged.

The parent who becomes single by divorce or death of a spouse is different from the unwed mother, for she or he has to overcome a crisis later in the family life cycle. Both parent and children experience this kind of crisis quite strongly and are very much in need of support from other people to overcome the emotional trauma. A nurse can be quite effective as a friend, if the client is willing to share and the nurse offers the time and support. The single parent's later ability to handle developmental stages depends to a great extent on how the initial crisis is handled. Nurses in this situation need to be concerned about parent and child's self-esteem, how they relate to each other, and how openly they communicate their feelings to each other.

Most single parents are also providers, although some are initially on public support. When the child goes to school, they may try to find a job to improve the family's lifestyle, but working outside the family may be an advantage or a problem, depending on the circumstances. While working mothers in nuclear families feel themselves burdened by increased responsibility, stress, and a lack of personal time, this is even more the truth for the single mother, with no husband to rely on for help with housecleaning, cooking, and so on. Many single women, however, become quite resourceful in establishing networks of mutual friends on whom they can count for favors. Some single-parent clubs operate with these objectives in mind and are a valuable help to single parents comfortable working within a friendship group.

Single fathers differ in the type of adjustment they have to make. Whereas they may have a more stable and secure economic base than a woman, they still must assume sudden responsibility for the family, housekeeping duties, hiring of babysitters, and so on. This burden may be very stressful for a father who does not have the resource of an extended family or a network of friends.

The advantage of mothers working is the necessity for their children to become independent and to hold their own. A well-functioning family usually maintains good communication, concern for each other, and the willingness to help out so that all gain a sense of needing and being needed. This sense of responsibility may be advantageous during teenage years, for it provides direction and purpose for the young person.

Families need to be evaluated individually, however, since other working mothers may feel guilty about being divorced and have the urge to make up to the children for what they had to suffer. As a result, they may not place enough restrictions on the children to avoid supposedly burdening them with responsibilities, and consequently may fail to meet their own needs.

Whether the step of letting the children go is hard or easy for a single parent cannot be determined without a look at other variables involved. If a single mother or father has been successful in a career and has been able to become established at work and in the community, church, and school, the step will be relatively easy. The variables operating here are the same as in the nuclear family, as are the tasks each individual must accomplish in later life; the only exception is that of having to maintain meaningful relationships outside the marriage rather than with a spouse.

The Extended Family

This type of family, a functional structure in rural settings but an economic liability within urban boundaries, is the norm in many cultures. Today some people have attempted to return to a lifestyle that includes group support, mutual acceptance, and affection and have embarked on experimental family adventures such as communes or religious communities. However, whether the family consists of a kinship group or a group of families held together by mutual agreement, the effect is basically the same. Since there are numerous adults responsible for the functioning of the family, the individual's responsibility is diminished. In order to function, a large group needs more structure, more rules and regulations, so that it becomes a community system in itself. Usually a leader emerges who is willing and able to take on the responsibility for the group as a whole. In the kinship family, the leader is often an older individual who is no longer providing but has the wisdom and knowledge to guide the others. Most communes do not last because of weak leadership and insufficient cohesion. In order for a group to function, it needs more direction toward a specific goal, and the goal must be the same for all members. Individual differences of values and opinions may prove destructive to the family system.

The primary difficulty, therefore, rests in the relationships between the members, which are much more complex than in the nuclear family, since more than two individuals are involved and they may have different backgrounds and values. The task of building up relationships and a system that is orderly, productive, and happy can be compared to the married couple stage in Duvall's (1977) framework for the nuclear family. The task is more difficult but essentially equal for the extended family if subsequent developmental stages are to be mastered, but instead of two people having to agree on how to raise the children, the decision must be made by all members.

In the extended family, children are not just the responsibility of the parents. In kinship families, the children are often raised by the older generation in order to free the younger people to work. Extended families that have developed their values over generations and that have strong emotional ties can provide a shared responsibility system that functions very well. Within the extended system less independence is required of the nuclear family; the larger family can be supportive, and stress is shared so that it affects each individual less. In addition, the children are helped in their later development, especially in the adolescent stage, and they form bonds of affection with several members in the family, so that the parent-child relationship is less intense and children feel part of the family as a whole. In the old family system, sons were not required to separate from the family, and daughters were welcomed in a new kinship group and were equally supported if they fulfilled their task of bearing children. Adolescence, therefore, was a less stormy and traumatic experience.

Aging within the extended family may be a rewarding process to all members, provided the elderly are given status and are recognized as political or spiritual leaders or looked up to for their experience and knowledge. If this is not the case, they may feel as useless as the elderly in the nuclear family. In the nuclear family, the ideal aging process previously described happens only if strong kinship ties are maintained even though the children live elsewhere. However, in a well-functioning extended family, fulfilled old people are the rule rather than the exception.

In a kinship group, the sense of sameness and of oneness develops naturally over time. In arbitrarily composed family groups, the same cooperation and cohesion usually remains utopian, for the individualistic nature of the people, their sense of competition for leadership, and their lack of submission to a common goal create friction within the system. Communication is also extremely hard to maintain without anger and hostility becoming part of it, and the tension and conflicting values make children confused. The dynamics then resemble those of a child torn between conflicting parents, although here they may learn to associate with or avoid several family members.

The blended family has similar problems. This family, composed of two remarried single parents and their children, also experience competition for power, mainly among the children. It is difficult for a parent to accept fully the partner's children and not favor his or her own. This demands a maturity that many such parents do not have, especially if they rushed into another marriage because they felt emotionally hurt and needed the security of a spouse and family. The ideal gets destroyed quickly after the person realizes the extent of the stress involved in a struggle among incompatible family members. Still, many blended families are successfully able to establish a positive relationship, affection for each other, and support and effective communication.

In short, whereas the extended and blended family systems that function have many advantages for the children as well as for adult members, today it is extremely hard to maintain or form an extended family group held together by nonconflicting relationships.

Many nuclear families enjoy some of the advantages of the extended family because strong kinship ties are maintained, even though the various generations may reside in different locations. Frequent visits and activities for the total family, sharing of children between members of different age groups, and mutual respect and affection lead to a system that relieves the nuclear couple of some responsibility, provides support, and gives the older generation a sense of being needed.

The community nurse should have a good understanding of the ideal family situation and the components needed to make it work. A family's strengths can then be used to improve what is already present for increased satisfaction of all members.

The Family Without Children

In 1976, 15 million people were living alone, according to Epstein (1980:81), and this number is growing. In addition, many more single adults were sharing the same household, and more married couples had decided not to have children. Such families do not have to be concerned about the development of growing children, but they too have tasks that, if not mastered, will lead to loneliness and despair.

Like the parents in the nuclear family, the relationship between adults in a family without children needs to deepen over time. A young, active couple with many outside interests may be able to meet both members' needs, but when illness strikes and emotional as well as physical support is needed, such relationships are put to the test. Institutions are filled with people who have lost their partners and who had failed to maintain close ties with children or friends and so found themselves alone.

In today's mobile society, stable support systems are not easy to build and maintain for the adult without kinship ties. During their younger years, people may be occupied with career, recreational, and other goals, and in old age despair over the lost mate or best friend may close the gates to the outside world.

The functional individual is able to build and maintain relationships intimate enough to permit sharing of feelings with others in the household or with friends outside. Often such relationships are transitory, and a person needs to dissolve old relationships and build new ones. Real intimacy develops over time, and frequent disruption of relationships can turn out to be detrimental. Since dissolving a relationship often leaves one with a feeling of loss, a person may try to protect himself or herself from future hurt of a loss in another relationship by avoiding getting involved with other people. Such coping may be effective protection, but it does not fulfill the individual's emotional needs. Other factors may also interfere with one's ability to form intimate relationships, such as psychological problems. Children who have not been accepted within their parents' family and have not formed strong attachments to their parents may have difficulties later in life in forming bonds with other persons. In addition, they are likely to lack the role models of their parents or other close persons. Today's pace of life, general superficiality of social interactions, and lack of concern of people in the community for each other may further contribute to the difficulties of people without strong family ties.

Nevertheless, community nurses may encounter many living arrangements that are satisfactory for all family members involved. Older individuals may share a household and find new joy and fulfillment with the help of each other, homosexual couples may live in a satisfactory relationship of mutual understanding and support, and young people may experience life's trials and rewards together as friends or by maintaining an informal sexual relationship. Again, the nurse's criteria for assessment of the family's functioning should not be related to the structure of the family but to the effectiveness of the means the individuals have found to satisfy their personal needs and maintain mutually gratifying relationships. At times, these relationships can be continued and deepened until the family members reach old age, but often an individual will need to engage in many different relationships until a final stability can be achieved later in life. Nurses can be helpful by alerting clients to their needs and by showing them ways in which they can get involved with other people like themselves. Often such persons need to learn to appreciate themselves and their own potential before they can overcome their depression and loneliness, and nurses may be a significant help in getting them started in recognizing their strengths and potential.

CONCLUSION

Throughout this book, we have stressed the holistic aspects of community nursing care, trying to guide the nursing student so that he or she will be able to render nursing care in ways that are richer, fuller in content, and more effective in assessing family needs as well as in the teaching of health principles. To accomplish this, we have outlined procedures for applying the nursing process to community health and for viewing clients as being shaped and influenced by their families and communities. This approach has translated theory into nursing action and interpreted the role of the community health nurse in the three aspects of care—primary, secondary, and tertiary prevention. Since understanding the nature of families and their dynamics and interaction with the environment is of prime importance for comprehensive nursing care, this topic has been explored extensively.

REFERENCES

Duvall EM: *Marriage and Family Development.* Philadelphia, Lippincott, 1977.
Epstein L: *Helping People: The Task-Centered Approach.* St Louis, CV Mosby, 1980.
Erickson E: *Childhood and Society,* ed 2. London, Hogarth Press, 1950.
Kahn MW: *Basic Methods for Mental Health Practitioners.* Cambridge, Mass, Winthrop Publishers, 1981.

Index